World Health Organization
Regional Office for Europe
Copenhagen

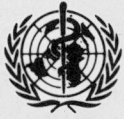

Management of drinking problems

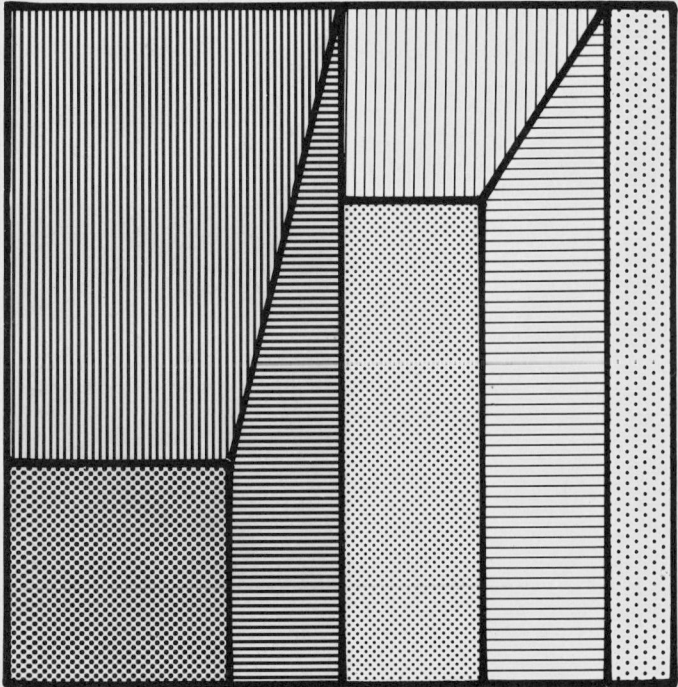

WHO Regional Publications, European Series, No. 32

The World Health Organization is a specialized agency of the United Nations with primary responsibility for international health matters and public health. Through this Organization, which was created in 1948, the health professions of some 165 countries exchange their knowledge and experience with the aim of making possible the attainment by all citizens of the world by the year 2000 of a level of health that will permit them to lead a socially and economically productive life.

The WHO Regional Office for Europe is one of six regional offices throughout the world, each with its own programme geared to the particular health problems of the countries it serves. The European Region has 31 active Member States,[a] and is unique in that a large proportion of them are industrialized countries with highly advanced medical services. The European programme therefore differs from those of other regions in concentrating on the problems associated with industrial society. In its strategy for attaining the goal of "health for all by the year 2000" the Regional Office is arranging its activities in three main areas: promotion of lifestyles conducive to health; reduction of preventable conditions; and provision of care that is adequate, accessible and acceptable to all.

The Region is also characterized by the large number of languages spoken by its peoples and the resulting difficulties in disseminating information to all who may need it. The Regional Office publishes in four languages — English, French, German and Russian — and applications for rights of translation into other languages are most welcome.

---

[a] Albania, Austria, Belgium, Bulgaria, Czechoslovakia, Denmark, Finland, France, Federal Republic of Germany, Greece, Hungary, Iceland, Ireland, Israel, Italy, Luxembourg, Malta, Monaco, Netherlands, Norway, Poland, Portugal, Romania, San Marino, Spain, Sweden, Switzerland, Turkey, USSR, United Kingdom and Yugoslavia.

Management of
drinking problems

WHO Library Cataloguing in Publication Data

Management of drinking problems

(WHO regional publications. European series ; no. 32)

1.Alcohol drinking 2.Alcoholism — prevention & control
3.Community health services 5.Europe
I.Series

ISBN 92 890 1123 8   (LC Classification: HV 5275)
ISSN 0378-2255

World Health Organization
Regional Office for Europe
Copenhagen

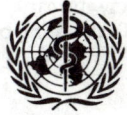

WHO Regional Publications, European Series, No. 32

Management of drinking problems

by

Peter Anderson

Director, National Unit for
Health Promotion in
Primary Health Care
Churchill Hospital
Oxford, United Kingdom

ICP/ADA 031
Text editing by Diana Gibson

ISBN 92 890 1123 8
ISSN 0378-2255

PRINTED IN DENMARK

CONTENTS

Introduction

In many parts of Europe alcohol consumption has increased considerably during the last 25–30 years. Simultaneously there has been a huge increase in alcohol-related problems, which are now regarded by a number of European countries as a major public health problem, second only to cigarette smoking (1,2).

Alcohol services have tended in the past to provide sophisticated specialist treatment for the few patients who either could afford to pay or lived near cities — but clearly the response to drinking and its consequences cannot come just from health workers. It is also quite unrealistic to expect any country to produce a group of specialists concerned solely with recognizing and treating these problems. WHO emphasizes the importance of a response embedded in the community (3) and the need for early recognition, and has also suggested ways of using reporting systems or other strategies for small-scale monitoring and evaluation (4,5). These strategies imply that early recognition is possible, and that nipping the problem in the bud will prevent further damage.

There is now increasing evidence that such strategies are justified. Nevertheless, careful evaluation of health promotion and simple intervention studies must continue, and more evidence of their efficacy is required. The logic and economic practicality of primary-level intervention is undisputed. However, more work is urgently needed to translate the rhetoric into workable, everyday activities. WHO has recently published a manual for community health workers on dealing with drug dependence and alcohol-related problems, which includes a set of guidelines for trainers (6).

This book aims to take these issues further and examine them in more detail. It is based on the reports of three working groups convened by WHO. The first group considered treatment and rehabilitation programmes for alcohol abuse (7). It concluded that in most European countries alcohol-dependent people place a heavy burden on society in terms of individual suffering, harm to others and high expenditure for

1

health and social services. But it also recognized that far more widespread damage may be done by the much larger percentage of people with high or even moderate levels of alcohol consumption, who may never reach the stage of alcohol dependence and whose physical, mental and social problems and their repercussions on the community go unrecognized and untreated.

In its report, this working group emphasized that the situation cannot be alleviated merely through recourse to long-term institutional care for people labelled as "alcoholics". In addition to major efforts aimed at the prevention of alcohol-related problems, there is an outstanding need for the recognition of incipient alcohol problems and for intervention starting at an early stage. This work can only be undertaken with the collaboration of personnel in the primary health care services. Their willingness and ability to do it, however, is generally impeded by their lack of training and by the inadequacy of assessment and intervention techniques for use in primary health care.

The second working group examined the respective roles of primary health care and specialized services in the development and implementation of programmes for problem drinkers (8). It concluded that there should be a redistribution of resources, emphasizing the role of primary care in the identification and management of individuals with drinking problems. This redistribution would depend on a community and political will that could be expected only from a population enlightened as to the nature of alcohol-related problems. This in turn implied an investment in health education in order to create a background of information from which responsible attitudes towards health and health promotion could develop. In the longer term, the group thought it likely that specialist services will take on a different role. If this happens then specialist personnel will help in making the transition to a more consultative and educational role, less identified with the institutional setting.

The third group reported on the implementation and evaluation of programmes for problem drinkers (9). It concluded that the risk factor approach — in which alcohol is viewed as a risk factor for social, psychological and physical ill health — should be adopted in the training and work of primary health care personnel. The services provided in a community should reflect that community's needs. In particular, services should be provided for moderate and heavy drinkers as well as for people with really severe drinking problems. This would require better coordination and joint planning by primary health care and specialist services.

The main body of this book follows the logical sequence of a strategy for the prevention and management of alcohol problems in primary care. Chapter 1 examines the part played by alcohol and drinking in communities and in individual lives. The risk to health from alcohol varies according to the level of consumption, the pattern of consumption and the time it has taken to reach that level. Each individual's consumption is the

2

result of a balance between factors that encourage drinking and those that discourage it; Chapter 2 discusses this balance and how it varies over a lifetime. In so far as they are rational and have access to good information, people are autonomous and can choose their own lifestyles and habits.

Chapter 3 catalogues the harm that can result from the use of alcohol in terms of social, psychological and physical functions; the extent of the damage done varies according to levels of consumption. This chapter also emphasizes that efforts to reduce the "moderate" drinking of the majority of patients will have a greater effect on the total health of society than similar efforts to reduce the consumption of those already damaged by alcohol.

Chapter 4 discusses the resources available for preventing and managing alcohol problems. There are four levels of care: self-care, informal care, primary health care, and care by specialist services. Only a minority of individuals with alcohol-related problems reach the secondary care level. Chapter 5 lists ways of promoting health and preventing alcohol problems. An ecological approach is recommended and ways are proposed of influencing both national and local decisions.

Chapter 6 suggests a structure for ascertaining and categorizing the alcohol-related risks for individuals seen in primary health care. After assessment, they can be placed in one of three categories, which will help determine the action needed. Chapter 7 discusses this action and suggests ways of informing, advising and helping both the large majority of patients in primary health care who will make minimal demands on staff time — those with low or intermediate level of consumption — and also the remainder, whose management will require the combined resources of primary health care staff, the patient's family, and outside bodies. It is emphasized that these demands are no different in scale or scope from those in other areas of clinical management such as raised blood pressure, sexual problems or the early detection of cancer.

The staff of primary health care services will need training to carry out the tasks outlined in the proposed strategy: they must be flexible in their methods, alert to the needs of the community, and ready to work with and learn from other professional and lay people. Chapter 8, therefore, discusses the entire sequence of education and training, ranging from undergraduate education through general and higher professional training to continuing medical education in practices and local communities. This education and training needs to be firmly grounded in facts determined by audit and research. Learning, audit and research should merge imperceptibly into each other and in turn form the basis of policies for prevention, screening, assessment and management.

1

What we drink

Alcohol consumption has roughly doubled in a number of European countries in the last 25 years. From 1960 to 1972 world production of beer increased by 68%, spirits production by 61% and wine production by 19% *(10)*. Since that time, consumption has continued to increase in most European countries with the exception of France and, more recently, Sweden.

Recorded Consumption

Because of tax and excise, many countries have good records of national alcohol consumption *(11–15)*. Routine national data are available for trade, production and consumption.

Table 1 presents the figures for European Community trade in alcoholic drinks between 1965 and 1985. Community trade in alcohol has expanded with increased membership, but it has also grown steadily between periods of accession. Intra-Community trade imports of wine increased despite low consumption levels in new member states, more than replacing imports from the rest of the world. The growth in intra-Community beer imports between 1970 and 1975 was stimulated by the accession of Denmark, Ireland and the United Kingdom, all countries with a high per capita beer consumption. However, extra-Community beer imports more than doubled after 1975. The most dramatic trade effect was the increase in intra-Community imports of spirits after United Kingdom accession and the parallel decline in the imports of foreign spirits.

The export figures in Table 1 also reflect the rapid expansion of Community trade in alcoholic beverages. The European Community is now the world's largest wine producer with growing exports to non-member countries.

Table 1. European Community trade in alcoholic beverages, 1965 – 1985 (in thousands of kilograms)

Year	European Community[a]	Wines		Beer		Spirits	
		Intra	Extra	Intra	Extra	Intra	Extra
Imports							
1965	6	343 788	1 133 671	146 275	72 891	17 155	59 950
1970	6	759 782	1 108 171	222 493	88 297	50 745	127 961
1975	9	1 735 628	501 141	812 949	37 565	203 849	113 842
1980	9	1 836 820	532 583	871 067	49 507	296 357	105 658
1985	10	2 287 385	471 428	1 039 997	79 615	349 982	77 813
Exports							
1965	6	283 980	306 960	154 870	165 156	26 671	84 043
1969	6	416 560	348 539	198 051	196 640	49 548	108 687
1975	9	1 658 352	494 551	800 698	441 273	239 922	544 473
1980	9	1 911 341	928 845	827 930	555 896	341 456	629 595
1985	10	2 588 723	1 095 248	980 664	835 760	385 324	616 989

[a] Total number of European Community member states at the time.

Source: Houveel alkoholhoudende dranken vorden er in wereld gedronken? (14).

Data on beer, spirits and wine production are given in Tables 2–4. The Federal Republic of Germany and the United Kingdom are the main brewers, producing nearly 60% of total beer output in 1984. Although production has increased in major brewing states, the most rapid expansion has occurred in countries entering the Community as small brewers.

Community spirits production is dominated by the output of whisky from the United Kingdom and of brandy and aniseed products from France and the Federal Republic of Germany. Production of spirits increased in all member states between 1970 and 1980, particularly in countries with low production levels.

Most European Community wine is produced in France, the Federal Republic of Germany and Italy. Total Community wine production increased steadily from 1961 under the Wine Programme. However, output has declined since 1980 in countries that produce mainly table wines. About 70% of all wine produced in the European Community is table wine.

Table 2. Beer production in the European Community, 1965–1984
(in thousands of hectolitres)

Country	Year				
	1965	1970	1975	1980	1984
Belgium	11 092	13 015	13 797	14 291	14 311
Denmark	4 655	7 087	9 039	8 169	8 499
France	19 795	20 255	22 316	21 684	20 288
Germany, Fed. Rep. of	73 170	87 051	93 457	92 342	92 583
Greece	530	779	1 377	2 500	2 829[a]
Ireland	4 159	5 040	6 120	6 000	5 423
Italy	4 558	5 959	6 463	8 569	9 141
Luxembourg	499	541	805	729	630[b]
Netherlands	5 402	8 724	12 434	15 684	17 048
United Kingdom	48 433	55 148	64 566	64 830	60 105
EC 10[c]	172 293	203 599	230 374	234 798	230 857
Portugal					3 665
Spain					21 833

[a] Estimate of Greek production at 2 829 — Dutch Distillers.

[b] 1983 figure — Dutch Distillers.

[c] European Community of ten.

Source: Powell *(15).*

Table 3. Spirits production in the European Community,
1970 to 1982/1983
(in thousands of hectolitres of pure alcohol)

Country	Year			
	1970	1975	1980	1982/1983
Belgium	52	61	80	79
Denmark	48[a]	63[a]	68[a]	94
France	2 100	2 819	2 830	1 781
Germany, Fed. Rep. of	1 198[a]	1 339[a]	1 342[a]	1 061
Greece	49[a]	83[a]	119[a,b]	—
Ireland	93	88	208	117
Italy	660	822[a]	923[a]	684
Luxembourg	—	—	—	1
Netherlands	274	461	419	331
United Kingdom	4 180	4 446	4 907	3 305[c]
EC 10[d]	8 495	10 185	10 898	—
Portugal				89
Spain				1 150

[a] Actual pure alcohol content unspecified; assumed an average strength of 35% alcohol.

[b] 1979 figure.

[c] 1983/1984 figure.

[d] European Community of ten.

Source: Powell *(15).*

Data on alcohol consumption have been used as major indicators of the need for government alcohol control policies across the world. The changing pattern of alcohol consumption in various European countries is shown in Table 5. A general trend towards more homogeneous consumption can be seen after 1960. Those countries recording the lowest levels of per capita consumption for any type of drink show the fastest growth in consumption. Per capita consumption of beer and spirits has grown in all countries, but wine consumption has decreased in the two main wine-producing nations, France and Italy. Disparity between the countries has declined, with an overall increase in alcohol consumption.

Per capita consumption data are derived from statistics produced by member states on volume sold or released for consumption. The data do

Table 4. Wine[a] production in the European Community, 1961 – 1984
(in thousands of hectolitres)

Country	Average over 4 wine years			Wine year	
	1961/1965	1971/1975	1976/1980	1980/1981	1983/1984
Belgium	4	6	4	4	2
France	60 594	68 278	67 699	69 598	67 523
Germany, Fed. Rep. of	5 184	8 222	8 315	4 867	13 000
Greece	—	5 115	5 366	5 395	4 734
Italy	62 253	69 561	74 024	83 950	81 848
Luxembourg	135	145	93	50	185
United Kingdom	—	1	2	2	11
EC 10[b]	128 170[c]	152 328	155 503	163 866	167 303
Portugal					8 300
Spain					30 400

[a] Production of all wines of various quality before distillation into wine alcohol.

[b] European Community of ten.

[c] European Community of six only.

Source: Powell *(15)*.

9

Table 5. Per capita alcohol consumption (in litres)
in the European Community of ten, 1960–1984

Country	Drink[a]	Year			
		1960	1970	1980	1985
Belgium	B	112.0	132.4	131.3	121.0
	W	7.8	14.2	20.6	22.7
	S	0.8	1.3	2.4	2.1
Denmark	B	71.4	108.5	121.6	121.2
	W	3.1	6.0	14.0	20.7
	S	0.6	1.3	1.5	1.6
France	B	35.3	41.3	44.3	40.1
	W	126.9	109.1	91.0	80.0
	S	2.0	2.3	2.5	2.3
Germany, Fed. Rep. of	B	95.7	141.14	145.7	145.5
	W	10.8	17.2	25.5	25.6
	S	1.9	3.0	3.1	2.4
Greece	B	5.5	9.4	26.3	33.9
	W	40.8	40.0	44.9[b]	42.5[b]
	—	—	0.6[b]	1.3[b]	1.3[b]
Ireland	B	67.3	100.6	121.8	108.4
	W	2.0	3.3	3.6	3.5
	S	0.8	1.5	2.0	1.8
Italy	B	5.1	11.3	16.7	21.6
	W	108.3	113.7	92.9	84.8
	S	1.0	1.8	1.9	1.2
Luxembourg	B	116.4	127.0	114.4	120.0
	W	31.4	37.0	48.2	57.3
	S	1.0	1.9	9.0	8.0
Netherlands	B	23.8	57.4	86.4	84.5
	W	1.9	5.2	12.9	15.0
	S	1.1	2.0	2.8	2.2
United Kingdom	B	85.1	101.6	117.1	108.9
	W	1.6	2.9	7.2	10.0
	S	0.7	1.0	1.8	1.7

[a] B = beer, excluding ciders; W = wine and fortified wine; S = spirits as 100% alcohol.

[b] Minimum estimates.

Source: Powell (15) and Brewers' Society international handbook.

not record consumption of home-produced alcohol, duty-free purchases,
alcohol released from stocks, or the non-recorded beverages such as
ciders in France. They relate only to drinks recorded as wines, beers or
spirits, and therefore underestimate consumption. However, it is also

10

possible that some of the figures overestimate consumption by domestic populations. For example, in 1984 Luxembourg had the highest rate of spirits consumption per head of population in Europe. It is likely that this figure is vastly inflated by the large numbers of tourists and other visitors who purchase alcohol in Luxembourg every year.

The overall change in per capita consumption of pure alcohol must be calculated from bulk volume series by assuming average alcohol strengths. There are no consistent series estimating approximate strengths for beers, wines or spirits consumed in different countries. Series derived from production figures will not necessarily reflect the strength of drinks consumed in any country.

In some countries customs and excise data, which record for tax purposes the total amounts of beer, spirits and wines retained for consumption, are available for long periods of time. In the United Kingdom for example, customs and excise records have been collected with only brief interruptions since 1684. Fig. 1 (16) shows that the United Kingdom has had several waves of increased alcohol consumption in the past 300 years, and that the present rise is small compared to those of the 1750s and 1870s.

Unrecorded Consumption

Routinely collected production and tax data do not include data about unrecorded consumption of alcohol. There are three important reasons for documenting unrecorded consumption: first, to have complete statistical accuracy in total alcohol consumption figures; second, because variations in unrecorded consumption may indicate important changes in drinking patterns (an increase in the production of home-made wines or beers may point to a growth in domestic hobbies); and third, because unrecorded consumption is important for studies on the interaction between alcohol policies and public attitudes and behaviour.

The Social Research Institute of Alcohol Studies in Finland has documented unrecorded consumption in that country (17). Data were collected under four headings: unrecorded or home production, unrecorded imports, unrecorded consumption by alcohol industry employees, and consumption of non-beverage alcohol. The data came from five sources: government control and crime statistics on medicines, smuggled spirits, home-distilled liquors and denatured spirits; sales statistics on raw materials and supplies, such as yeast, distilling equipment, and crushed barley malt for home-made beer; estimates by experts; observations; and surveys. The findings are given in Table 6. The sum total of unrecorded consumption remained fairly constant throughout the study period of the 1950s to the 1970s. However, unrecorded consumption as a proportion of recorded consumption decreased, due to a huge growth in recorded consumption.

11

Fig. 1. Alcohol consumption in the United Kingdom, 1680–1975

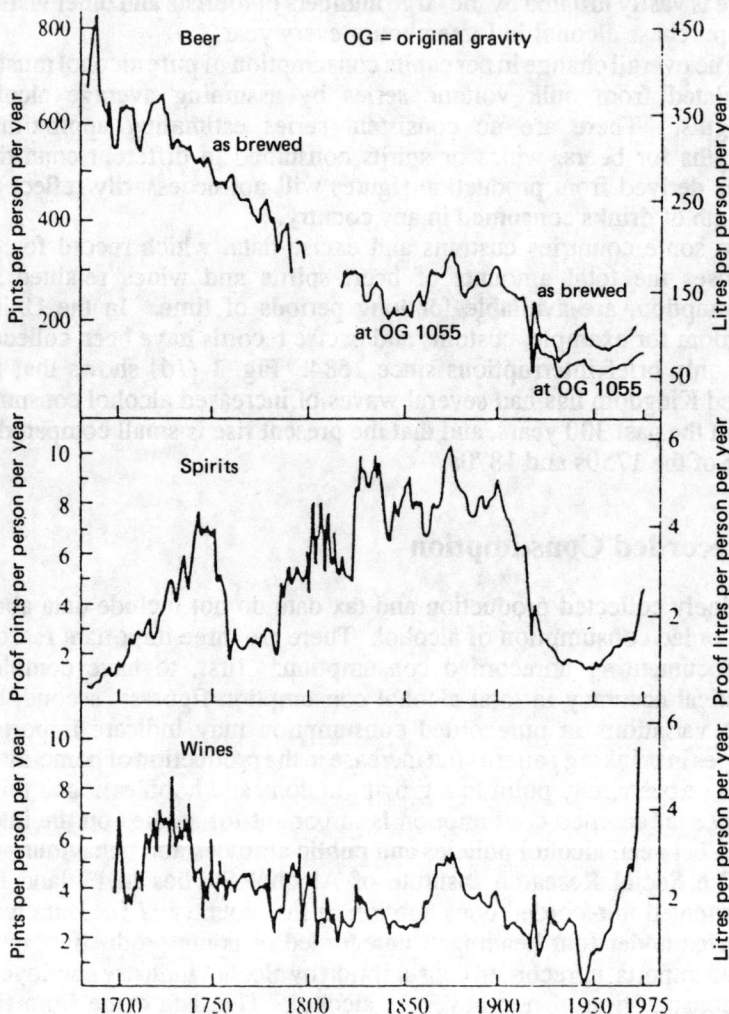

Source: Spring & Buss (16).

Routinely Collected National Data

In a number of countries government departments routinely collect data on alcohol use (18). In the United Kingdom, for example, there are two

12

annual surveys, the General Household Survey *(19)* and the Family Expenditure Survey *(20)*. The General Household Survey, conducted by the Office of Population Censuses and Surveys, has been running since 1971. Each year all adults (those aged over 16) in approximately 10 000 private households are questioned on core topics related to social policy. Questions on drinking, using a quantity frequency format, have been included biennially since 1978 (Table 7). The response rate is 82–84%.

Table 6. Unrecorded and recorded consumption of alcohol
in Finland in the 1950s, 1968 – 1969 and 1976

Item	Period		
	1950s	1968 – 1969	1976
Breakdown of unrecorded consumption (in litres of 100% ethanol)			
Sahti[a]	150 000	280 000	270 000
Kilju[b]	250 000	130 000	80 000
Home-made wines	400 000	400 000	400 000
Pontikka[c]	300 000 – 450 000	25 000	250 000
Imported by travellers	50 000 – 200 000	400 000	1 200 000
Smuggled alcohol	120 000 – 600 000	180 000	50 000
Consumed by alcohol industry employees	negligible	negligible	negligible
Medicines containing alcohol	400 000 – 500 000	negligible	negligible
Spiritus fortis[d]	?	75 000	75 000
Other rectified alcohol	?	?	?
Cosmetic products containing alcohol	80 00 – 120 000	negligible	negligible
Strongly denatured alcohol	50 000	280 000	negligible
Total unrecorded consumption	1 800 000 – 2 720 000	1 770 000	2 325 000
Recorded consumption (in millions of litres of 100% ethanol)	6.9 – 8.4	1968: 13.5 1969: 19.8	29.8
Unrecorded consumption as a percentage of recorded	21.4 – 39.4	1968: 13.1 1969: 8.9	7.8

[a] Traditional home-brewed beer.

[b] Sugar-fermented home-made alcohol.

[c] "Moonshine".

[d] Surgical and rectified spirits provided to pharmacists by Alko.

Source: Mäkelä *(17)*.

13

Table 7. Drinking habits in the United Kingdom,
1978 and 1982

Type of drinker[a]	Men		Women	
	1978	1982	1978	1982
	(%)	(%)	(%)	(%)
abstainer	5	6	11	12
occasional	9	10	25	23
infrequent light	11	12	19	20
frequent light	34	37	39	40
moderate	15	14	4	4
heavier	25	21	2	1
	(N)	(N)	(N)	(N)
Sample size (= 100%)	10 015	8 780	11 650	10 185

[a] Persons aged 18 or over only.

Source: Office of Population Censuses and Surveys (19).

The Family Expenditure Survey, begun in 1957, provides information on private households in the United Kingdom and their expenditure patterns. Responders keep a diary in which they make a detailed record of expenditure over 14 consecutive days, including spending on alcoholic drinks (Table 8). Some 11 000 households take part in the study, and response rates of 68–71% are achieved.

Ad Hoc Surveys

A number of countries obtain information on alcohol consumption from ad hoc surveys on either national or regional sampling frames (21–26). For example, random samples of the Dutch population of age 20 and over were interviewed in 1958, 1970 and 1981 on, among other things, alcohol consumption (26). Changes in the distribution of consumption in various subpopulations are shown in Table 9. Between 1958 and 1981 the increase in per capita consumption in the Netherlands was more than 300%. The surveys show that this increase in consumption was due neither to a decrease in the proportion of abstainers nor to a decrease in the differences in alcohol consumption between different subpopulations.

Tables 10 and 11 show drinking patterns in England & Wales for women and men, respectively. The results were obtained by detailed questioning about drinking during the week before interview (21). They

14

show that there are major differences between the amounts consumed by the two sexes, and it is younger adults, particularly young men, who are most likely to drink heavily. The survey also showed that there were no consistent variations in alcohol consumption between different social classes in England & Wales, although workers in the construction and drinks industries drank more than those in other industries. This study also demonstrated regional differences in consumption patterns, people in the north of the country being the heavier consumers.

It has been found that most drinking surveys cover only 40–60% of total alcohol consumption as indicated by taxation figures (27–30). There may be many reasons for this deficiency. For example, the validity of a survey may be undermined if it either misses or inadequately samples the target population. In many studies the pool of respondents is selected from electoral registers; heavy drinkers may cluster within certain districts, therefore the likelihood of their being sampled in a random survey is small. Moreover, drinkers of this type may live in institutions such as the armed forces, hospitals, prisons, colleges and so on, or they may be homeless; in neither case will they appear in the register.

It is also argued that the heavier drinkers included in a sampling frame are not only harder to locate but also more likely to refuse an interview. Various health and preventive studies in Scandinavia have compared participating and non-participating middle-aged men using data drawn from medical, police, forensic, temperance and taxation registers. These studies showed that non-participants had higher rates of alcohol-related morbidity and mortality and were more likely to be unmarried or divorced, and also poorer, than participants (31). However, it was shown that non-participants in a British survey who were later interviewed by post did not differ substantially from participants in either sociodemographic characteristics or self-reported consumption levels (32).

The respondent's forgetfulness about alcohol consumption increases or decreases according to the drinking measure used in the survey. Respondents tend to underestimate the frequency of their drinking, and to overestimate the quantity they have consumed on a typical drinking occasion. Several researchers have estimated memory loss for the week prior to interview by assuming complete recall of the previous day and comparing that answer with responses for the other days. Sixteen per cent of all drinking occasions were forgotten in a Canadian study (27), as were 9% of occasions and 8% of consumption in an English study (28).

Several studies have dealt with memory loss over longer periods. A Finnish study showed that estimates of daily consumption recorded in diaries over a period of six weeks were 60% higher than estimates given in answer to repeat questionnaires (33).

Deliberate underreporting of alcohol consumption may occur, because of the stigma associated with alcohol abuse and its behavioural effects. It seems to be particularly pronounced among respondents who are male, young and employed and among heavier drinkers. The extent

Table 8. Consumer expenditure in the United Kingdom, 1976–1984

	1976	1977	1978	1979	1980	1981	1982	1983	1984 Indices/ percentages	1984 Current prices (m£)
Indices at constant 1980 prices										
Food	97	96	98	100	100	99	99	101	99	28 448
Alcoholic drink	95	95	100	104	100	97	94	98	100	14 416
Tobacco	100	95	103	103	100	93	86	85	82	6 621
Clothing and footwear	85	86	95	101	100	99	103	110	116	13 158
Housing	92	94	95	98	100	101	103	104	106	29 239
Fuel and power	95	98	99	104	100	100	98	98	97	9 574
Household goods and services										
Household durables	94	88	94	105	100	98	101	109	112	7 016
Other	100	97	104	103	100	100	101	106	109	6 182
Transport and communication										
Purchase of vehicles	83	73	93	107	100	100	102	122	116	9 536
Running of vehicles	92	93	97	98	100	101	104	105	107	13 578
Other travel	90	90	93	98	100	100	96	99	106	6 457
Post and telecommunications	73	77	85	96	100	101	102	105	113	3 528
Recreation, entertainment and education										
TV, video, etc.	82	84	90	99	100	111	124	140	152	4 875
Books, newspapers, etc.	99	98	99	100	100	97	94	91	90	2 724
Other	88	91	96	99	100	99	98	99	102	10 157
Other goods and services										
Catering (meals, etc.)	97	99	98	101	100	92	91	98	100	11 048
Other goods	104	106	112	112	100	101	104	103	107	5 879
Other services	88	91	93	97	100	103	110	119	126	8 880

										£ million
Less expenditure by foreign tourists, etc. in the United Kingdom	107	122	114	110	100	91	89	96	102	4 866
Household expenditure abroad	53	51	63	80	100	106	106	107	106	4 224
Final expenditure by non-profit bodies	96	94	96	97	100	102	103	108	112	3 999
Consumer expenditure	91	91	96	100	100	100	100	104	106	194 673
Percentage of total consumer expenditure at current prices										
Food	18.4	18.6	18.0	17.2	16.7	15.9	15.4	15.0	14.6	28 448
Alcoholic drink	7.6	7.6	7.3	7.3	7.3	7.3	7.2	7.3	7.4	14 416
Tobacco	4.1	4.2	3.9	3.6	3.5	3.6	3.5	3.4	3.4	6 621
Clothing and footwear	7.7	7.7	7.9	7.8	7.2	6.7	6.6	6.6	6.8	13 158
Housing	13.4	13.4	13.2	13.2	13.7	14.8	15.5	15.0	15.0	29 239
Fuel and power	4.7	4.9	4.6	4.5	4.6	5.1	5.2	5.2	4.9	9 574
Household goods and services	7.6	7.3	7.6	7.6	7.3	6.9	6.7	6.8	6.8	13 198
Transport and communication	14.9	14.7	15.5	16.4	16.6	16.7	16.6	17.1	17.0	33 099
Recreation, entertainment and education	9.1	9.3	9.4	9.2	9.2	9.2	9.3	9.1	9.1	17 756
Other goods, services and adjustments	12.6	12.4	12.7	13.1	13.8	13.8	14.0	14.5	15.0	29 164
Total	100.0	100.0	100.0	100.0	100.0	100.0	100.0	100.0	100.0	194 673

Source: United Kingdom National Accounts, Central Statistical Office.

17

Table 9. Consumption levels of different Dutch subpopulations in 1958, 1970 and 1981 (percentages)

	1958					1970					1981				
	Ab-stainers	≤3 glasses	4–12 glasses	13–21 glasses	≥22 glasses	Ab-stainers	≤3 glasses	4–12 glasses	13–21 glasses	≥22 glasses	Ab-stainers	≤3 glasses	4–12 glasses	13–21 glasses	≥22 glasses
Sex															
Men	11.6	62.1[a]	19.3[a]	5.0[a]	2.0[a]	13.7	28.2[b]	33.5	13.9[b]	10.7[b]	13.2	20.3[c]	32.4[c]	18.3[c]	15.7[c]
Women	28.8[c]	65.2[a]	7.1[a]	1.8[a]	0.2	31.3	44.2[b]	19.0[b]	5.1[b]	0.7[b]	30.3	32.6[c]	26.1[c]	8.6[c]	2.4[c]
Men															
21–40 years	11.1	58.8[a]	22.1[a]	5.7[a]	2.3[a]	8.8	23.6	33.7	19.4	14.5	11.3	18.4[c]	35.3[c]	18.4[c]	16.6[c]
≥41 years	12.1[a]	65.1[a]	16.7[a]	4.3[a]	1.8[a]	19.8	33.3[b]	31.6	8.4[b]	6.9[b]	15.2	22.2[c]	29.5[c]	18.1[c]	14.9[c]
Women															
21–40 years	19.5	68.8[a]	10.3[a]	1.4[a]	—	22.8	42.4	27.6	6.2	1.0[b]	27.1[c]	36.7[c]	23.6[c]	9.0[c]	3.5[c]
≥41 years	30.7[a]	62.3[a]	4.6[a]	2.2	0.3	38.2	43.3[b]	13.6[b]	4.4[b]	0.5	33.7	28.2[c]	28.8[c]	8.0[c]	1.2
Men															
More educated	13.6[a]	60.5[a]	19.7[a]	4.8	1.4[a]	19.9	33.9[b]	28.3	8.7[b]	9.1	15.3	22.8[c]	30.6[c]	17.4[c]	13.9[c]
Less educated	9.2	63.9[a]	18.9[a]	5.2[a]	2.8[a]	10.5	15.4[b]	36.1	16.5	11.6[b]	11.6	18.4[c]	33.9[c]	18.9[c]	17.2[c]
Women															
More educated	28.9[a]	64.7[a]	4.4[a]	2.1	—	44.4[b]	41.1	11.1[b]	2.4[b]	1.0	35.2	35.5[c]	21.1[c]	6.5[c]	1.7[c]
Less educated	19.9	66.2[a]	12.1[a]	1.3[a]	0.4	22.6	46.2[b]	23.9[b]	6.8[b]	0.4	24.8	29.3[c]	31.8[c]	10.9[c]	3.2[c]

18

Men

No religious denomination	8.9	61.5[a]	23.7	5.2[a]	0.7[a]	14.0	26.1	31.3	15.0	13.7	13.2	20.2[c]	33.3[c]	16.9[c]	16.5[c]
Roman Catholic	9.1	59.8[a]	22.0[a]	5.4[a]	3.7[a]	13.2	23.7	33.8	16.9	12.4[b]	9.8	17.3[c]	31.6[c]	22.2[c]	19.1[c]
Protestant	16.0	67.9[a]	11.7[a]	3.7[a]	0.8[a]	13.7	34.9[b]	35.6	9.9	6.0	13.0	24.4[c]	38.2[c]	16.0[c]	8.4[c]

Women

No religious denomination	27.8	63.2[a]	7.6[a]	1.4[a]	0.0	27.9	42.3[b]	22.4	6.6	1.2	24.8	33.0[c]	30.3[c]	10.6[c]	1.4
Roman Catholic	22.0	67.5[a]	7.8[a]	2.2[a]	0.4	27.6	46.9[b]	18.8	5.9	0.8[b]	28.0	32.0[c]	27.1[c]	8.4[c]	4.4[c]
Protestant	27.8[a]	64.3[a]	6.2[a]	1.7	—	37.2	43.5	16.1	3.2[b]	—	35.2	32.4[c]	22.5[c]	7.7[c]	1.6

Men

(Total: 2035)	171	337	63	27	11	117	242	287	119	92	84	129	206	116	100

Women

(Total: 2095)	433	47	12	1	238	338	145	39	5	202	217	174	57	15

[a] Significant difference between 1958 and 1970.

[b] Significant difference between 1970 and 1981.

[c] Significant difference between 1958 and 1981.

Note. Two-sided *t*-test significant at $P \le 0.05$.

Source: Knibbe et al. (26).

19

Table 10. Alcohol consumption in the previous week, by age,
in England & Wales — females

Type of consumption	Age group (years)					
	18-24	25-34	35-44	45-54	55-64	≥65
	(%)	(%)	(%)	(%)	(%)	(%)
Nondrinker	5	6	8	8	11	24
Occasional drinker (nothing to drink in previous week)	17	25	27	33	41	39
1-5 units	38	41	38	33	33	25
6-10 units	12	11	13	10	7	6
11-20 units	18	14	10	12	7	4
21-35 units	6	2	2	3	1	1
36-50 units	—	1	1	1	—	—
51-75 units	2	—	1	—	—	—
76 units or more	2	—	—	—	—	—
	100	100	100	100	100	100
Sample size	125	222	179	157	158	221

Source: Wilson (21).

of underreporting is influenced by specific aspects of the interview, including the characteristics of the interviewee (30).

Underreporting may also occur when the questions are inappropriate. In a Finnish study higher consumption estimates were obtained from alcohol-dependent individuals when questions focusing on high consumption were used in place of questions concerning low or moderate consumption which were normally used for non-dependent respondents (34).

* * *

Although drinking surveys underestimate the total amount of alcohol consumed, therefore, when compared to taxation figures, the biases are likely to be consistent over time, so that surveys do allow the study of changes in drinking patterns and of differences between the various age and sex groups. The next chapter examines the reasons behind an individual's drinking level.

Table 11. Alcohol consumption in the previous week, by age,
in England & Wales — males

Type of consumption	Age group (years)					
	18-24	25-34	35-44	45-54	55-64	≥65
	(%)	(%)	(%)	(%)	(%)	(%)
Nondrinker	2	5	5	4	10	9
Occasional drinker (nothing to drink in previous week)	5	7	13	19	22	37
1-5 units	13	18	18	21	25	21
6-10 units	14	16	14	16	11	9
11-20 units	17	20	21	15	13	13
21-35 units	25	15	15	11	9	8
36-50 units	11	10	9	10	6	2
51-75 units	8	5	6	4	3	1
76 units or more	5	3	1	1	1	—
	100	100	100	100	100	100
Sample size	123	177	151	166	143	173

Source: Wilson *(21).*

21

Why we drink

In recent years a new framework has been developed, by the British Psychological Society *(35)* in particular, for understanding the reasons why people drink certain amounts. According to this framework, drinking is seen as spread along a continuum, from harmfree drinking at one end to harmful drinking at the other. An individual's drinking behaviour is learned and modified by experience; at any stage it is determined by a balance of the advantages and disadvantages, the pleasure and the harm. All drinkers, whatever their current level of drinking, also have the choice of moving forward or backward along the continuum.

If a cross-section of people, including those who are concerned about their drinking and those who are not, are asked why they drink, they will give a very mixed bag of answers *(36)*:

to feel more relaxed in company	to relieve a hangover
because it goes well with meals	to perform sexually
to make me feel more relaxed	to have a good laugh
to pick me up when I feel tired	to get drunk
to help me go to sleep	to feel good
to relieve a stressful situation	only because I'm offered a drink
at home	because it's the social custom
I like the taste	for no particular reason
to relieve boredom	I wouldn't miss it if it wasn't
to quench my thirst	there

There may also be deeper reasons which are not so easily recognized or expressed:

to reduce threats to one's	to achieve peer status
feelings of adequacy	to relieve role-strain in one's
to protect against depression	job
to relieve internal conflict	to enhance fantasies of personal
prompted by one's dependence	power
on alcohol	as self-reward

to express rebellion against parents or others in authority	as self-punishment
	as sedation
to ease the tensions of an unhappy home life	to relieve sex-role conflict

These lists are incomplete, but their length and variety illustrate a number of things. First, like other drugs and activities that can be used for psychological purposes — such as eating or gambling — alcohol can serve a wide variety of functions *(37)*. Taken in different doses and consumed over varying periods of time, it can have very different psychopharmacological effects. Furthermore, it is so widely available in so many different forms that its use can change according to the concentration of alcohol in a particular drink, the time of day, the company in which it is drunk, the place where it is drunk, and the meaning of the occasion (a celebration, a negotiation, a last fling, a drink before a meal, and so on). Not only this, but its effects also depend on personality and on an individual's expectations. Experiments have shown that, at least in moderate doses, whether a drink produces laughter, sexual arousal or further drinking depends not on what it contains but on whether the consumer was told that it contained alcohol *(38)*. Hence, as with all psychoactive drugs, expectation plays a role.

Incentives

Given this variety of functions that alcohol can serve and the complexity of its psychopharmacology, it is no surprise that different people derive different kinds of benefit from it, depending upon their age, sex, stage in their life cycle and role. The same substance that among young people can serve to increase social confidence, enhance status among friends, give the courage to rebel, and relieve boredom or sexual anxiety can help a middle-aged professional man to face the stresses brought about by an unhappy marriage, rebellious children, a tiring, highly stressful and frustrating job, or feelings of mortality and mid-life crisis. Women who drink in a way that puts them at risk are less likely than their male counterparts to refer to the positive social functions of drinking and more likely to refer to the strains and role conflicts of being wives and mothers or the tensions of combining responsibilities inside and outside the home *(39)*.

It is important to remember that the determinants of drinking behaviour are as much social, cultural and environmental as they are personal. Almost all surveys of the drinking behaviour of young people find that involvement in drinking is correlated with the behaviour of their friends. The peer group appears to be the single most important determinant at least of early drinking patterns in adolescence and young adulthood *(37)*. (The same is true for cigarette smoking and the use of other drugs.)

Drinking is largely a social and recreational activity, so it is understandable that friends have a major influence on drinking habits, and not only in the case of young people. Women in particular continue to be highly influenced by the drinking practices of their male companions, and it is known that the husbands of women who drink excessively or harmfully are likely to be heavy drinkers themselves (40).

Although excessive drinking may become a solitary affair for some people later on in their lives, for most people — and particularly for men — drinking remains a social phenomenon for most of their drinking careers. It is more the rule than the exception to find in the drinking histories of excessive drinkers that some period has been spent living or working in an environment where alcohol was more than usually readily available, and where heavy drinking was the norm (41). Not only are individuals at risk because of the personal functions that heavy drinking may serve for them, but certain environments are risky for the individuals who inhabit them. For example, life in France carries a higher risk of cirrhosis of the liver than life in Norway (Fig. 2). In the United Kingdom, entering adulthood in the early years of this century was more risky in terms of drinking than immediately after the Second World War (Fig. 3). Being brought up in England by first-generation Irish immigrants is riskier than being brought up in England by indigenous English parents (43). Working in a brewery or a public house is riskier than being an accountant (Table 12).

On this last point, there are clear links between alcohol-related problems and occupation. In the United Kingdom, for example, publicans have a mortality rate from cirrhosis of the liver of 15 times the average, and fishermen 6 times. The reasons for these differences lie within the realms of easy availability of drink, its relative cheapness, social pressures to conform, separation from normal social and family restraints, opportunities for unsupervised drinking, stress, and also the selection and self-selection of high-risk individuals. In England & Wales the construction industry had the highest proportion (19%) of men drinking over 50 units weekly (21), compared to only 6% in this category in the male population as a whole. Men in the drinks industry had the highest consumption per person employed — 38 units weekly, compared to 20 units weekly for the whole male population.

In recent years awareness has also grown that risky drinking is not just a matter of individual psychology or pharmacology or occupation, but also of public health. There is a direct relationship between public controls of alcohol consumption such as price manipulation on the one hand, and overall consumption of alcohol and rates of alcohol-related problems on the other. National consumption and death rates from cirrhosis of the liver, for example, are highly correlated (1). There is also considerable evidence that the whole drinking continuum in a population can be shifted by external factors such as price increases and availability.

25

Fig. 2. Alcohol consumption and death rates from cirrhosis of the liver in selected countries (mid-1970s)

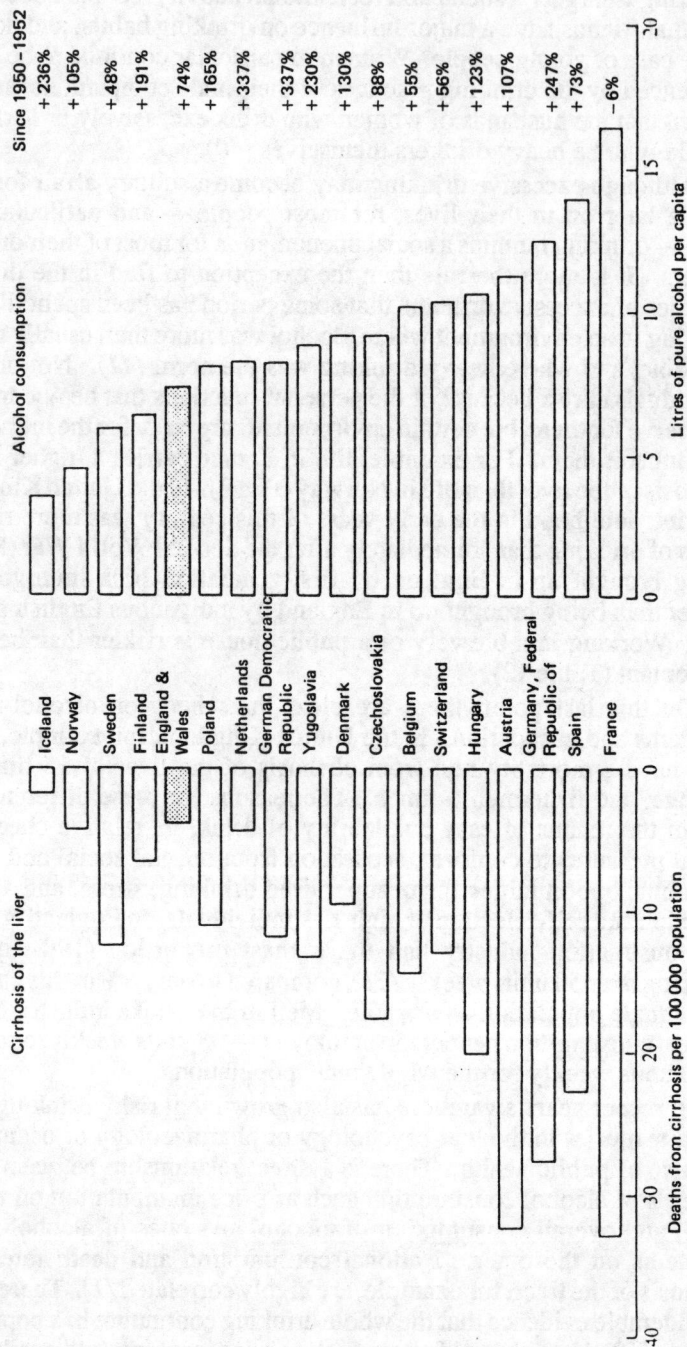

Cirrhosis of the liver

Alcohol consumption

Since 1950–1952

Country	Since 1950–1952
Iceland	+236%
Norway	+105%
Sweden	+48%
Finland	+191%
England & Wales	+74%
Poland	+165%
Netherlands	+337%
German Democratic Republic	+337%
Yugoslavia	+230%
Denmark	+130%
Czechoslovakia	+88%
Belgium	+55%
Switzerland	+56%
Hungary	+123%
Austria	+107%
Germany, Federal Republic of	+247%
Spain	+73%
France	–6%

Litres of pure alcohol per capita

Deaths from cirrhosis per 100 000 population

Source: *Alcohol — reducing the harm (42)*.

Fig. 3. Alcohol consumption by type, United Kingdom, 1900–1984

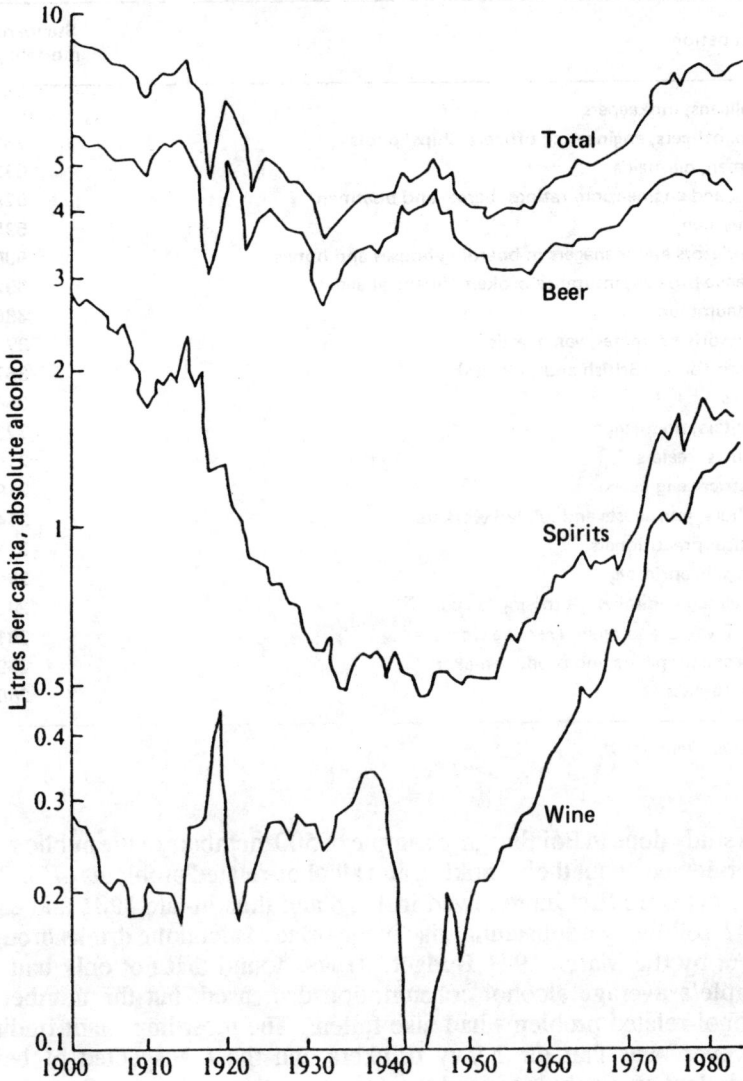

Source: Alcohol — reducing the harm (42).

Table 12. Mortality from liver cirrhosis in England & Wales, 1970-1972

Occupation	Standardized mortality rate
Publicans, innkeepers	1576
Deck officers, engineering officers, ships' pilots	781
Barmen, barmaids	633
Deck and engine-room ratings, barge- and boatmen	628
Fishermen	595
Proprietors and managers in boarding-houses and hotels	506
Finance brokers, insurance brokers, financial agents	392
Restaurateurs	385
Lorry drivers' mates, van guards	377
Armed forces (British and overseas)	367
Cooks	354
Shunters, pointsmen	323
Winders, reelers	319
Electrical engineers	319
Authors, journalists and related workers	314
Medical practitioners	311
Garage proprietors	294
Signalmen and railway-crossing keepers	290
Maids, valets and related service workers	281
Tobacco preparers and product-makers	269
Metallurgists	266

Source: Plant *(44)*.

In a study done in Edinburgh, a sample of 500 members of the public were interviewed about their drinking and alcohol-related problems *(45)*. The subjects were first interviewed in 1978 and then in late 1981 and early 1982, following a substantial rise in the price of alcoholic drinks brought about by the March 1981 Budget. It was found that not only had the sample's average alcohol consumption decreased, but the number of alcohol-related problems had also fallen. The most important finding, however, was that the heavy drinkers and those suspected of being dependent on alcohol reduced their consumption just as much as people who drank more moderately.

A part of the answer to the question of why people drink, then, is that people are subject to a variety of individual and social factors that influence their disposition to drink. Some people are affected by factors such as cultural background, peer group, occupation, stress, genetic makeup and so on that put them at risk of drinking much or drinking often (the two are not necessarily the same, since drinking patterns vary) whilst others are affected by factors that put them at much lower risk.

Disincentives

There is one important respect in which the picture given so far is incomplete. It shows only the attractions or incentives for drinking, and has nothing to say about the restraints, the disincentives, the reasons why individuals do not drink, or do not drink more than they do. There are a whole host of disincentives or discouragements that influence people's drinking behaviour. These include unpleasant physiological responses to alcohol: there is evidence, for example, that some Orientals have an unpleasant flushing response to quite small doses of alcohol (46). Other disincentives may be financial restraint, lack of time and effort to devote to drinking because of preoccupation with other interests and activities, disapproval by family, friends or colleagues, a philosophical preference for an aesthetic rather than a hedonistic way of life, or membership of religious, cultural or other groups that proscribe the excessive or even any use of alcohol. Some people may never have been exposed to the use of alcohol, or not have learned to drink during their upbringing.

Reinforcing Influences

The framework for understanding drinking is made all the more complicated by the fact that human beings and their motivations rarely stand still, but are subject to change and development during the course of a lifetime. One study of the development of young adults' drinking behaviour over a four-year period gives a good example of this (47). It was found that whether a young person was a drinker or not was correlated with a number of factors, including the person's conformity or non-conformity, and the number of close friends who were drinkers. These factors were not simply causal factors, however. They changed over a period of four years, as did the drinking: the young people who became less conformist and more likely to be drinkers were also more likely to have friends who drank, as time went on. Furthermore, it was also shown that becoming a drinker at a particular stage was associated with a reduction in conformity both before and after the onset of drinking. This study shows that a change in behaviour such as drinking does not occur in a psychological vacuum, but as part of a group of changing beliefs, preferences and habits, and that drinking behaviour cannot be divorced from the demands, both biological and social, of particular stages in the life cycle.

Plant's study of the drinking habits of employees in the drinks trade (41) demonstrates the same point. Plant was interested to know whether being employed in this trade was risky in terms of drinking because of factors inherent in the job, or whether it was a matter of self-selection, with people who were already heavy drinkers opting to enter that environment. In fact, it turned out to be both. As a group, people who enter the drinks trade are heavier drinkers than others, but they also become heavier drinkers still, once they are on the job.

Both the students in the first study and employees in the second were subject to a process of positive feedback. The older the students became, or the older the employees were on entering a new job, the more likely they were to drink. The more likely they were to drink, the more they lost their innocence. The more they lost their innocence, the more likely they were to drink.

There are a number of other developmental processes that have a great deal to do with the development of habitually excessive or risky drinking. One of these is the process of learning, whereby behaviour that is rewarded or reinforced sufficiently often becomes habitual and difficult to eradicate. This process is much aided by conditioning, whereby formerly neutral stimuli such as the sights and sounds of a public house or cafe, the smell of a favourite drink, and all the paraphernalia associated with a pleasant drinking occasion take on emotionally positive connotations because of their associations with the rewarding results of drinking. The whole process may then be bolstered by positive mental images or thoughts such as "What I really need now is a good drink"; "I'm a real man if I can hold my drink"; or "People who don't drink heavily are boring". These processes in combination are immensely powerful (47).

Other reinforcing processes take effect in later stages of the drinking career. One is the development of an altered psychobiological response to drinking. Increased tolerance, the presence of withdrawal symptoms when blood alcohol levels fall, and the discovery that the malaise can be relieved by further drinking, create an additional source of motivation for regular and excessive drinking that makes the habit more difficult to break. Increased tolerance to the effects of alcohol is acquired as a result of a history of drinking. It relates to the amount drunk and the length of time drinking. It is acquired gradually, is relatively greater for some functions and abilities than for others, and may be reduced during periods of abstinence or much lighter drinking. Both increased tolerance and withdrawal symptoms which may be relieved by further drinking are sometimes quite rapidly reinstated, within a few days, if drinking is resumed after a period of abstinence or lighter drinking. This increased tolerance should not be confused with reduced (or reversed) tolerance, which usually develops after a much longer history of risky drinking. Then, quite moderate levels of drinking may give rise to much greater than usual effects and damage, probably because of brain and/or liver damage. The late stages of a long drinking history may also be complicated by some degree of cognitive impairment caused by damage

30

to the central nervous system, which can then affect the ability to make choices about future drinking.

There are social and personal processes that have the same effect. Increasingly heavy drinking may tend to lead a person towards the company of other heavy drinkers, and away from the company of moderate drinkers. It may lead the individual to seek employment in which drink is more easily available. Some of the harmful effects of excessive drinking such as losing a job, or becoming estranged from family, may themselves cut the person off from some of the major constraints to heavy drinking. The loss of self-confidence and self-respect and the increase in worry and tension often associated with heavy drinking themselves add weight to the pressure towards heavier drinking.

Moderating Influences

As well as these reinforcing processes, there exists a parallel set with a moderating effect. The financial burden of heavy consumption, for instance, may cause the drinker to cut back on drinking; or the awareness that it is affecting work may lead to a resolve to drink less or not at all for a period. Advice that gastritis and overweight are in large part attributable to excessive drinking may help a patient to take immediate corrective action; or again the realization that their drinking is getting out of control induces some people to seek expert advice.

The role of the family in moderating drinking cannot be overemphasized. Particularly for people who live in a family setting — and this includes the majority of excessive drinkers — the family plays a major part in helping or hindering the achievement of a lower level of drinking. By encouraging excessive drinking, or unwittingly contributing to a downward spiral of increased family tension and disengagement, a family may make it more difficult for one of its members to drink less. On the other hand, the family may become the principal cause for change by influencing the drinker in favour of moderate drinking, and by continuing to give constructive care and affection (48).

An important implication of the argument developed in this chapter is that no fundamental difference exists between spontaneous and therapeutic improvement. There is good evidence that people with alcohol problems often treat themselves and can move away from harmful alcohol use by drinking less. Vaillant, for example, reported the results of a longitudinal study of 456 Boston boys aged 14 years who were followed up for 35 years from 1940 (49). During this period 110 of them developed symptoms of alcohol abuse, but 48 of these subsequently achieved at least one year of abstinence, and 22 were able to return to social drinking. About one third of the 48 who became abstinent and 9 of the 22 who returned to social drinking did so with the aid of professional treatment, and about one third of the abstainers had also been

helped by Alcoholics Anonymous. Most, however, helped themselves.
A number of factors enabled these subjects to become abstinent: in
particular, 48% of them had developed a medical problem that was
instantly made worse by further drinking and so reminded them con-
stantly of the need to change their drinking habits.

* * *

An individual's position, then, on the continuum which runs from
abstinence at one end to excessive and risky drinking at the other depends
on the balance struck between a whole host of factors, some of which
incline towards drinking and others that restrain it. For every individual
there is an attraction/deterrence equation that determines drinking behaviour. Another way of expressing this is to say that everyone has a balance
sheet with entries on one side representing factors that incline him or her
to drink or to drink more, while the entries on the other side incline the
person to drink less (Tables 13 and 14).

Table 13. Hypothetical balance sheet of a moderate drinker

	Pay-offs from drinking	
	Positive	Negative
Feelings	"High", stimulated after a few drinks	Headache, dry mouth and mildly depressed next morning if I have drunk a lot
Performance	Increased energy and motivation immediately after lunch	Reduced concentration at work in the afternoon if I drink at lunchtime
Relationships with others	Closer, less tense with work colleagues	—
Economic	—	Leaves money short at the weekend if I drink a lot on Friday night
Other	Part of enjoyable relaxation at snooker club and at home with family and friends	—

Source: Robertson et al. (35).

32

Table 14. Hypothetical balance sheet of a heavy drinker

| | Pay-offs from drinking | |
	Positive	Negative
Feelings	Helps cope with family and job worries, relaxes	Feel guilty about drinking so much
Performance	Can face working after a few drinks	Making mistakes at work; one or two near-misses in car
Relationships with others	Meet several other heavy drinkers in the local who are good company; able to assert myself	Family complaining about not seeing me much; have embarrassed them a few times; they say I'm a changed character after drinking
Economic	—	Can't afford what I'm spending on drink
Other	—	I've put on a lot of weight

Source: Robertson et al. *(35)*.

It is within this framework of a balance sheet of advantages and disadvantages of drinking and a continuum along which an individual may move, forwards or backwards, at different stages of life that the primary health care worker's role can be considered. Being uniquely well placed and well qualified to detect signs of risky and harmful drinking and to influence those who are drinking to excess, primary health care workers have a crucial role to play.

3

Damage

In recent years there has been a fundamental reappraisal of the nature of the damage done by alcohol. The old belief, that "alcoholics" were different from the rest of the drinking population and the cause of society's problems, has been replaced by the idea that drinking and the harm done by it range along a continuum from minimum alcohol consumption with little damage and slight risk, to heavy consumption with a high probability of damage and high risk. So, broadly speaking, alcohol can be seen as a risk factor. Anyone who drinks is at risk, but by and large the more alcohol consumed, the greater the risk. In this respect alcohol is similar to blood pressure and serum cholesterol, both of which range from low to high and are risk factors for ill health. The higher the level of blood pressure the greater the risk of cerebrovascular disease, and the higher the serum cholesterol level the greater the risk of coronary heart disease.

National Data

A large amount of data is collected routinely on indicators of alcohol-related damage. Mortality data, collected from death certificates written by attending physicians, include mortality from cirrhosis and other alcohol-related conditions as well as from alcoholism and alcoholic psychosis. These data vary considerably in both accuracy and the recording rates for alcohol-related conditions on death certificates. It is possible that incorrect entries are common, due either to negligence or to diagnostic error. For example, ischaemic heart disease may be recorded instead of cardiomyopathy of alcoholic origin, and conditions related to chronic alcoholism are sometimes omitted. Such figures, important though they are, are not enough to show the scale of the problem. Excessive drinking is a contributory or determining factor in many diseases or deaths attributed to other causes such as cancer of the upper

35

respiratory tract, the digestive system and the oesophagus, or deaths in road and industrial accidents.

Other routinely collected data include hospital admissions for conditions such as liver cirrhosis, alcoholism, alcoholic psychosis and intoxication, and data on charges for drunkenness and drinking-and-driving. Some countries routinely collect data for both hospitals and primary care services.

Many of these data are also collected on a regional basis. However, it can be very difficult to interpret regional differences in damage indicators. In the United Kingdom, for instance, many indices of alcohol problems show regional variations, with higher figures in the north of England and in Scotland than in the south (50,51). Part of the difference can probably be attributed to differences in detection, recording and the provision of services (52–54).

The consumption/damage relationship

The idea that alcohol consumption and damage are related had its origin in the work of Ledermann (55). He made two assertions: first, that in a homogeneous population the distribution of alcohol consumption is a log-normal curve (Fig. 4), and second, that the number of people who drink a certain amount can be calculated if the average consumption is known. Although Ledermann's work, which is essentially theoretical, has been severely criticized and is the subject of much debate (56–58) nevertheless the curves of distribution of alcohol consumption produced by various surveys in different countries, although not exactly log-normal, are similar and are always skewed and unimodal (59,60).

The evidence that consumption and damage are related depends less on theory than on empirical evidence, however. Because of tax and excise, many countries have good records of national alcohol consumption. They do not record home-made alcohol, but until recently in most countries this was only a small part of total consumption. Some countries also have systems of death certification going back over 100 years. Putting together the figures for consumption and damage produces striking correlations that convince most people of the link between the two. Table 15 gives figures for consumption and alcoholic deaths in Britain for five-year periods from 1885 to 1934 (61). The correlation is clear. More recent evidence both from England & Wales (Table 16) and Finland (11,62) (Table 17) links consumption not only with alcoholic deaths but also with convictions for drunkenness, hospital admissions for alcoholism, drunken driving, alcohol-related accidents and crimes of assault. The comparison of alcohol consumption and deaths from cirrhosis in various countries (Fig. 5) provides further evidence of the link between consumption and damage (42). There is also some evidence, supported by surveys, that an increase in consumption will produce a disproportionate increase in damage. An increase in consumption of 50% between 1965 and 1974 in the Camberwell district of London was

36

Fig. 4. Ledermann's hypothetical curve

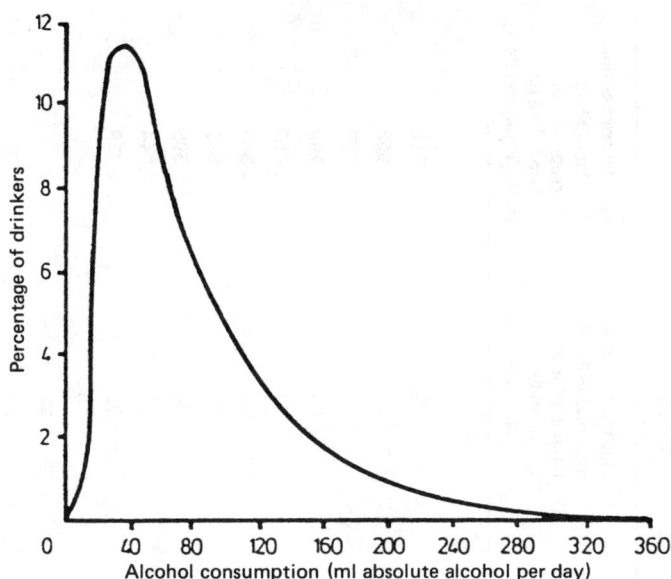

Table 15. Alcohol consumption per capita and number of deaths certified as being due to cirrhosis, delirium tremens or chronic alcoholism in the United Kingdom, 1885–1934

Five-year period	Average annual consumption (in litres of proof spirit)	Average annual number of deaths per million population
1885–1889	17.3	154
1890–1894	18.2	168
1895–1899	19.1	182
1900–1904	18.6	193
1905–1909	16.4	156
1910–1914	15.5	131
1915–1919	10.5	81
1920–1924	10.5	59
1925–1929	9.1	55
1930–1934	7.3	42

Source: Royal College of Psychiatrists *(61).*

37

Table 16. Alcohol consumption, convictions for public drunkenness, cirrhosis deaths and alcohol-related hospital admissions in England & Wales, 1950–1976

Year	Annual per caput consumption of persons aged 15 and over in litres of 100% ethanol	Convictions for public drunkenness per 10 000 population aged 15 years and over	Cirrhosis deaths with and without mention of alcohol per million population	Hospital admissions with primary diagnosis of alcoholism or alcoholic psychosis
1950	5.2	14.0	23	
1951	5.3	15.8	25	512
1952	5.3	15.8	26	668
1953	5.1	15.7	26	775
1954	5.2	15.5	26	799
1955	5.3	15.8	26	1 053
1956	5.3	17.4	26	1 385
1957	5.3	19.3	27	1 535
1958	5.3	18.7	26	1 595
1959	5.6	18.6	27	2 044
1960	5.8	19.3	28	2 479
1961	6.2	21.0	30	
1962	6.1	23.3	28	
1963	6.2	22.8	28	
1964	6.5	21.0	28	5 423
1965	6.5	19.8	29	5 774

Year				
1966	6.5	19.0	29	6 088
1967	6.7	20.3	28	6 232
1968	7.0	21.2	30	6 391
1969	7.0	21.2	32	6 689
1970	7.3	21.6	28	8 091
1971	7.7	22.9	32	9 230
1972	7.7	23.7	34	10 167
1973	7.9	25.9	37	11 565
1974	8.9	26.8	36	12 495
1975	9.4	27.0	37	12 751
1976	9.7	28.0		

Source: Royal College of Psychiatrists *(61).*

39

Table 17. Alcohol consumption per capita, arrests for drunkenness, crimes of assault and battery, cases of drunken driving, alcohol-related traffic accidents, deaths from liver cirrhosis and deaths from alcohol poisoning, per 100 000 population in Finland, 1950 –1975

Year	Consumption in litres of 100% ethanol	Arrests for drunkenness	Crimes of assault and battery	Cases of drunken driving	Alcohol-related road traffic accidents	Deaths from liver cirrhosis	Deaths from alcohol poisoning
1950	1.73	3668	148		20		2.2
1951	1.79	3349	148	37	21	2.3	2.5
1952	1.87	3387	145	50	25	2.5	2.5
1953	1.85	3222	139	50	24	2.4	2.1
1954	1.88	3030	142	46	25	3.2	2.5
1955	1.97	3070	133	43	25	3.3	2.8
1956	1.83	2927	123	49	24	3.0	3.1
1957	1.72	2923	121	49	23	3.5	3.0
1958	1.62	2763	119	58	23	3.6	2.7
1959	1.72	2947	127	75	27	3.2	2.4
1960	1.85	2964	125	96	28	3.3	2.9
1961	2.01	3157	126	116	35	3.5	2.9
1962	2.11	2933	125	119	40	3.4	2.4
1963	2.17	3049	120	128	42	3.5	2.7
1964	2.21	2916	119	135	48	3.5	3.0
1965	2.35	3029	126	144	51	3.4	3.0
1966	2.49	3157	131	152	51	3.2	

Year							
1967	2.64	3337	139	154	46	3.2	4.8
1968	2.88	3185	155	147	45	3.6	5.2
1969	4.21	2966	212	178	53	4.1	4.3
1970	4.30	3722	237	197	59	4.2	4.6
1971	4.72	4415	251	215	64	4.1	4.9
1972	5.10	4421	265	243	70	4.3	5.0
1973	5.60	4920	279	289	78	4.5	3.7
1974	6.45	6098	289	350	77	5.4	5.5
1975	6.19	5842	277	379	75	6.3	4.3

Source: Österberg (11).

41

Fig. 5. Liver cirrhosis death rates and alcohol consumption in various countries in the mid-1970s

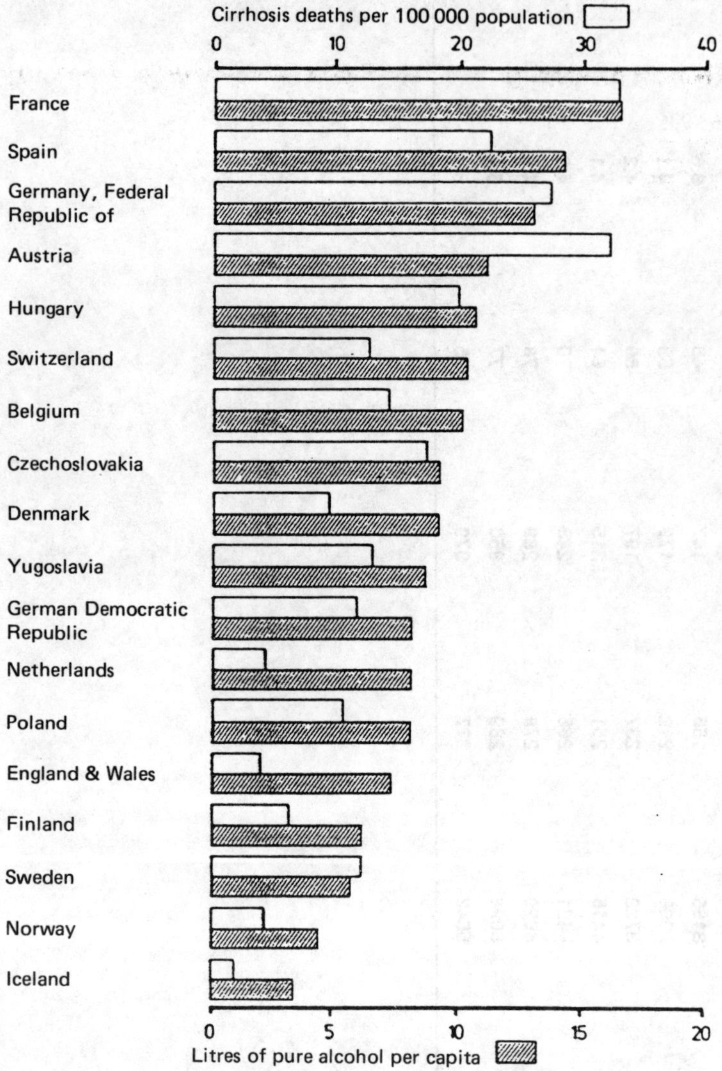
Cirrhosis deaths per 100 000 population
0
10
20
30
40
France
Spain
Germany, Federal Republic of
Austria
Hungary
Switzerland
Belgium
Czechoslovakia
Denmark
Yugoslavia
German Democratic Republic
Netherlands
Poland
England & Wales
Finland
Sweden
Norway
Iceland
0
5
10
15
20
Litres of pure alcohol per capita

Source: *Alcohol — reducing the harm (42).*

associated with a threefold increase in the number of people falling into the highest drinking categories *(63)*.

The general rule that consumption is related to damage continues to apply in smaller groups, but the pattern is not so neat. A study of four

Scottish towns — Inverness, Aberdeen, Glasgow and Ayr — found that although the towns with the higher consumption had more damage, there were exceptions to the general rule *(60)*. First, the town with the highest average consumption, Inverness, did not have as many "heavy" heavy drinkers as Glasgow. This was partly explained by Glasgow having the most abstainers. Second, small variations in consumption were associated with large variations in problems. For example, average consumption in Inverness was only 49% higher than in Ayr, and yet crime rates were more than 1000% higher, hospital admission rates were about 800% higher, and mortality was twice as high. Many factors must be involved in explaining these differences. Consistent heavy drinking every day, as in France, gives high cirrhosis rates, while "binge" drinking", as in Inverness, leads to more problems associated with drunkenness.

There is good evidence linking changes in alcohol consumption with changes in alcohol-related disorders. The relationship between alcohol consumption and deaths from cirrhosis is clearly established *(64)* (Fig. 6). In the United Kingdom, the cirrhosis death rate rose by 3% a year from 23 per million in 1950 to 44 per million in 1979. The relationship also holds good over time, in regions in other countries, from one country to another *(65)*, and for other causes of death, including causes related to intoxication *(66–68)*.

Furthermore, when alcohol consumption decreases, so does the number of problems (Fig. 7). In the year 1981–1982, for the first time in postwar Britain, consumption of alcohol fell, from 10.4 litres of pure alcohol per adult to 9.2 litres. This fall was associated with an 11% reduction in convictions for drunkenness, an 8% fall in drinking-and-driving convictions, and a 4% fall in deaths from liver cirrhosis *(69)*.

Similar relationships between declining alcohol consumption and alcohol-related problems have been observed in other countries. In Sweden, for example, sales of alcohol dropped 17% from 1976 to 1982 *(70)*. Mortality from cirrhosis of the liver declined between 1979 and 1982 by 28% in men and 29% in women (Fig. 8). During the same period mortality from pancreatitis declined by 30% in men and 36% in women. The decline in alcohol-related problems was greatest among young people *(71)*. Analysis of county figures confirm these changes. In Stockholm County a computer-based inpatient care register has covered 97–99% of all hospital discharges since 1973. This has made it possible to study the utilization of inpatient care and mortality simultaneously in a metropolitan area during a period of decreased alcohol sales. Between 1976 and 1984 in Stockholm County there was a 20% fall in the sale of alcohol. Over the same period there was a decline in inpatient care for liver cirrhosis and pancreatitis for both sexes, and in alcoholic psychosis, alcoholism and alcohol intoxication for men. The mortality for liver cirrhosis and pancreatitis also dropped, and there was a levelling-off of mortality due to alcoholic psychosis, alcoholism and alcohol intoxication.

Fig. 6. Deaths from alcoholism and cirrhosis.
Offences for drunkenness and consumption of alcohol in England & Wales, 1860–1978

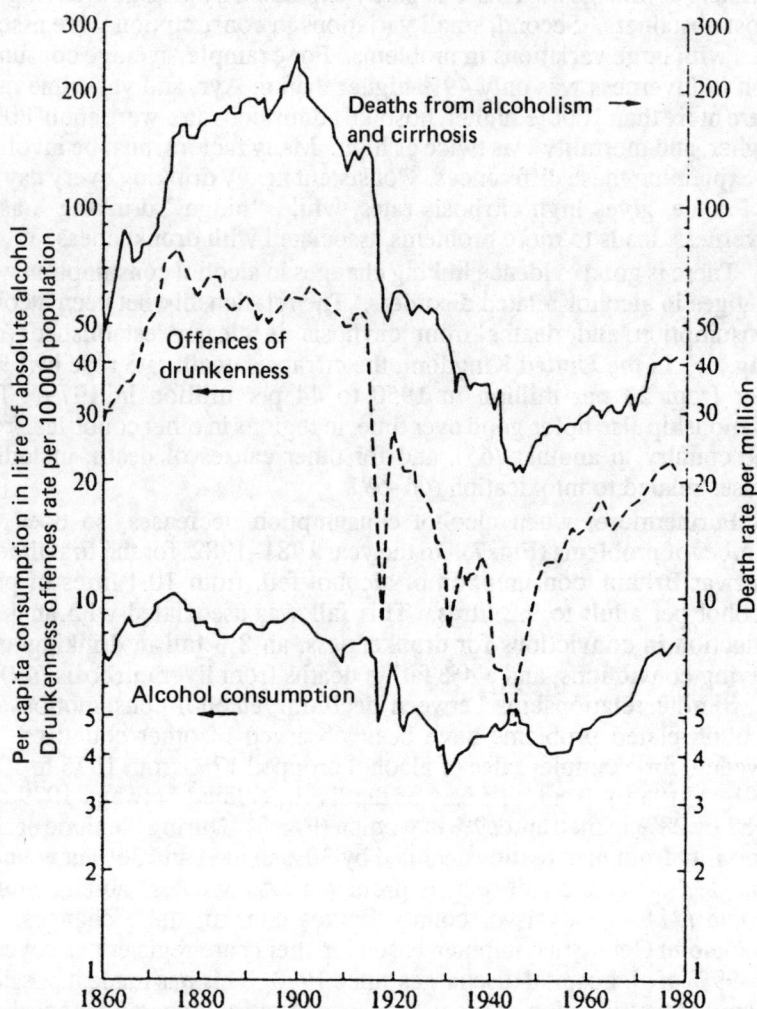

Source: Alcohol — reducing the harm (42).

Social cost

The overall cost of alcohol consumption to any society will be determined by a number of factors. Included in this are the total amount of alcohol consumption and the patterns of drinking. In England & Wales

Fig. 7. Alcohol consumption, drunkenness convictions, alcoholism admissions and cirrhosis mortality, 1970–1982 (all per person aged 15 or over)

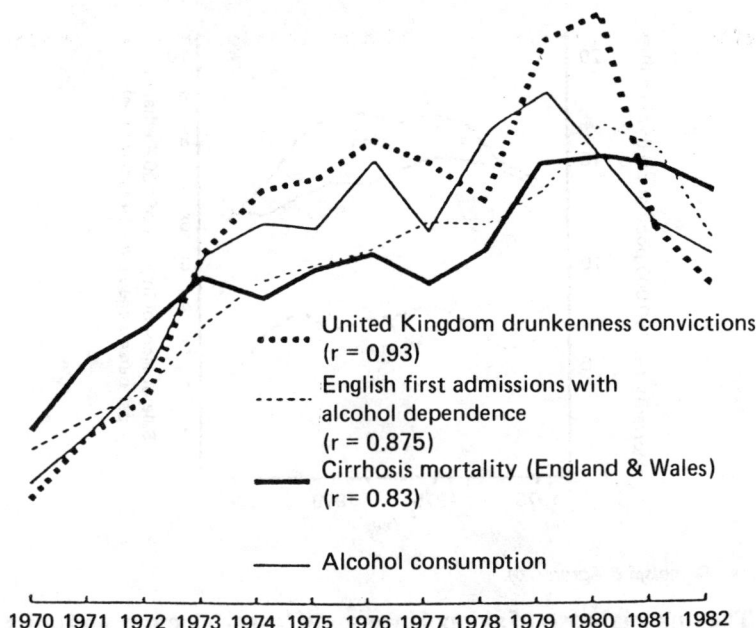

United Kingdom drunkenness convictions
(r = 0.93)

English first admissions with
alcohol dependence
(r = 0.875)

Cirrhosis mortality (England & Wales)
(r = 0.83)

Alcohol consumption

1970 1971 1972 1973 1974 1975 1976 1977 1978 1979 1980 1981 1982

Source: Kendell (69).

it has been estimated that 700 000 people (2% of the total adult population) have serious problems related to alcohol, and 3 million (8%) are heavy drinkers, drinking at levels leading to detectable biochemical abnormalities *(42)*. Heavy drinkers have a mortality rate over twice that of the normal population. In Britain, although only 3000 death certificates a year mention alcohol, the true premature mortality for which alcoholic intoxication or psychosis could be blamed is probably in the order of 5–10 thousand a year. In the Malmö Preventive Population Programme, which followed up a cohort of 7935 middle-aged men in Sweden for three to eight years, alcohol was the cause of death in 25% of the 218 premature deaths, compared with 28% due to cancer and 23% due to coronary heart disease *(72)*.

An estimate based on data published in 1976 concerning individuals in alcohol treatment units suggested that the excess mortality from alcohol in England & Wales was 8000 a year *(73)*. An updated suggestion based on population studies is that there are 40 000 deaths due to alcohol in the United Kingdom each year, compared with 100 000 deaths due to cigarette smoking (Table 18) *(74–85)*.

45

Fig. 8. Mortality from cirrhosis of the liver in Sweden, 1973–1982, by year and sex related to sale of alcohol in litres of 100% ethanol for each subject aged over 14

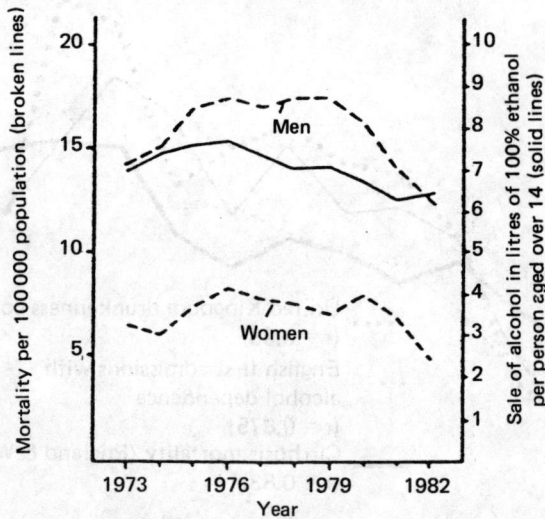

Source: Romelsjö & Agren (70).

The financial costs of alcohol in terms of lost production, and costs to the medical and social services in caring for individuals with alcohol problems, can be calculated. A conservative estimate for England & Wales gives the cost as at least £1600 million a year (Table 19) (85). Additional indirect costs, such as the costs of alcohol-related crime, fire and inefficient work in many fields, are hard to quantify.

A number of estimates have been made of the costs of alcohol consumption to the health services, although most of the figures used are recognized to be underestimates (86). A number of studies have shown that up to one in five patients admitted to medical wards in the United Kingdom have problems related to alcohol (87,88).

In addition to the workload for accidents, a Scottish study indicated that one in five male admissions to a general medical ward was related to the patient's use of alcohol (89). In another Scottish study 15% of female emergency admissions to a general medical unit were alcohol-related (90,91).

Individual Data

Before discussing individual types of damage related to alcohol use, it is necessary to consider the diagnostic classifications and terminology used

Table 18. Estimate of proportion of deaths attributable to alcohol, England & Wales, age 15+, 1984

	Percentage of deaths	
	Men	Women
Malignant neoplasms (ICD 140–239)	4	3
Cerebrovascular disease (ICD 430–438)	12	3
Respiratory disease (ICD 460–519)	11	2
Digestive disease (ICD 520–579, excluding 571)	12	3
Chronic liver disease (ICD 571)	80	80
Injuries and poisonings (ICD 800–899)	40	40
Other	6	1
All deaths	12	3

Source: Kagan et al. *(74,75)*, Kozarevich et al. *(76,77)*, Dyer et al. *(78,79)*, Rothman *(80)*, Holtermann & Burchell *(81)*, Adelstein & White *(82)*, Marmot *(83)*, Klatsky et al. *(84)*, McDonnel & Maynard *(85)*.

to describe alcohol-related disabilities. Both the concepts and the terminology have changed considerably over the last few years. For much of the first half of this century problems resulting from alcohol use were regarded as complications of a single disease — "alcoholism" — which was considered to have a predominantly genetic basis and a predictable natural history *(92)*. This concept of a disease has been criticized by many workers, who instead have favoured the idea that a complex of alcohol-related disabilities are associated with a certain level of alcohol consumption *(93,94)*.

The disease concept of "alcoholism" has been adopted particularly in North America. In 1980 the American Psychiatric Association, in their *Diagnostic and statistical manual of mental disorders*, made the distinction between "alcohol abuse" and "alcohol dependence". The criteria for alcohol abuse were three:

— continuous or episodic use of alcohol for at least one month;

— social complications of alcohol use; and

— psychological dependence (e.g. compulsion to drink) or pathological patterns of alcohol use, or both.

For a diagnosis of alcohol dependence, the additional criterion of either tolerance or experience of withdrawal symptoms was applied.

Edwards & Gross *(93)* took the converse approach in their description of the alcohol-dependence syndrome. They conceived the syndrome as being a psychobiological state characterized by a reorientation of life around alcohol, awareness of a compulsion to drink, and drinking to

47

Table 19. Total resource costs of alcohol misuse, England & Wales, 1983 prices

	£m
Social cost to industry	
Sickness absence	641.51
Housework services	42.23
Unemployment	144.74
Premature death	567.70
Social cost to the National Health Service	
Psychiatric hospitals, inpatient costs (alcoholic psychosis, alcohol dependence syndrome, non-dependent abuse of alcohol)	17.90
Non-psychiatric hospitals, inpatient costs (alcoholic psychosis, alcohol dependence syndrome, alcoholic cirrhosis and liver disease)	7.87
Other alcohol-related diseases inpatient costs	68.58
General practitioner visits	1.51
Society's response to alcohol-related problems	
Expenditure by national alcohol bodies	0.55
Research	0.49
Social cost of material damage	
Road traffic accidents (damage)	89.20
Social cost of criminal activities	
Police involvement in traffic offences (excluding road traffic accidents)	4.54
Police involvement in road traffic accidents (includes judiciary and insurance administration)	11.89
Drink-related court cases	15.79
Total (including unemployment and premature death)	1614.50
Total (excluding unemployment and premature death)	902.06

Source: McDonnel & Maynard *(85)*.

avoid the discomfort of its absence. They distinguished between this syndrome and the broader range of problems that result from harmful drinking, which were termed "alcohol-related disabilities" *(94)*. The crucial point is that both the alcohol-dependence syndrome and alcohol-related disabilities were considered to vary in their degree of severity.

The terms harmful alcohol consumption and hazardous consumption are relatively new, and are included in the provisional recommendations for classification in the Tenth Revision of the International Classification of Diseases. Harmful alcohol consumption denotes consumption that is causing harm to the psychological or physical wellbeing of the individual. Hazardous alcohol consumption is defined as a level of consumption or a pattern of drinking that is likely to result in harm, should present drinking habits persist.

There are two types of alcohol-related disabilities: disabilities relating to intoxication and disabilities related to regular heavy consumption (Tables 20 and 21). There is considerable overlap between the two tables. For example, both intoxication and regular heavy drinking are associated with a risk of stroke.

An important aspect of damage related to intoxication is that the population of individuals who suffer it is not static. Drinkers who are intoxicated on any one day will not necessarily be at risk of damage on a different day. It is likely that the majority of drinkers will at some stage of their lives experience some problems due to intoxication. The type and nature of the problems will vary from individual to individual, and also according to the circumstances in which the alcohol is drunk, for example when working or when driving.

For convenience, it is useful to consider alcohol-related damage under the three headings of social, psychological and physical. In reality, of course, an individual's experience may involve a combination of all three. Heavy drinking may lead to marital difficulties (social damage), which in turn may cause unhappiness (psychological damage). This may be followed by even heavier drinking, harming the liver (physical damage).

Social damage

The idea of social damage implies failure on the part of an individual to perform adequately in any role expected of him or her, for example in the family or at work. It may also include behaviour which transgresses social rules — crime, for example, or sexual deviance. Social damage, of course, depends very much on social norms, which may be different for men and women, for different age groups, for different social classes, and certainly for different countries.

Both intoxication and regular heavy drinking are associated with a wide range of problems involving families and children. Excessive drinking is a frequent cause of marital disharmony and divorce. In one study of 100 battered wives in the United Kingdom, 52 of the victims reported that their partners frequently drank heavily *(95)*. Financial stress will almost inevitably result from heavy consumption, affecting the wellbeing of the rest of the family. Children are especially at risk, and the results can be devastating *(96–98)*. Neglect is related to both intoxication and regular heavy drinking; the same may be true for child abuse *(99–101)*. Heavy drinking in one member of a family seems to impose a greater load of illness on others in that close environment.

An adverse impact on school work is common; in adolescence a son or daughter may be ashamed to invite friends home, so escapes by spending little time there. The emotional harm done in childhood can result in disabilities continuing into adult life *(102–104)*.

49

Table 20. Problems relating to intoxication

Social problems	Psychological problems	Physical problems
Family arguments	Insomnia	Hepatitis
Domestic violence	Depression	Gastritis
Child neglect/abuse	Anxiety	Pancreatitis
Domestic accidents	Amnesia	Gout
Absenteeism from work	Attempted suicide	Cardiac arrythmia
Accidents at work	Suicide	Accidents
Inefficient work		Trauma
Public drunkenness		Strokes
Public aggression		Acute alcohol poisoning
Football hooliganism		Failure to take prescribed
Criminal damage		medication
Theft		Impotence
Burglary		Fetal damage
Assault		
Homicide		
Drinking and driving		
Taking and driving away		
Road traffic accidents		
Sexually deviant acts		
Unwanted pregnancy		

Table 21. Problems relating to regular heavy drinking

Social problems	Psychological problems	Physical problems
Family problems	Insomnia	Fatty liver
Divorce	Depression	Hepatitis
Homelessness	Anxiety	Cirrhosis
Work difficulties	Attempted suicide	Liver cancer
Unemployment	Suicide	Gastritis
Financial difficulties	Changes in personality	Pancreatitis
Fraud	Amnesia	Cancer of mouth, larynx,
Debt	Delirium tremens	oesophagus
Vagrancy	Withdrawal fits	Cancer of breast (?)
Habitual convictions	Hallucinosis	Cancer of colon (?)
for drunkenness	Dementia	Nutritional deficiencies
	Gambling	Obesity
	Misuse of other drugs	Diabetes
		Cardiomyopathy
		Raised blood pressure
		Strokes
		Brain damage
		Neuropathy
		Myopathy
		Sexual dysfunction
		Infertility
		Fetal damage
		Haemopoietic toxicity
		Reactions with other drugs

People in certain occupations have exceptionally high rates of alcohol-related problems. High-risk jobs include those in the drinks trade, catering, the armed forces, the merchant navy, fishing and journalism. In all jobs excessive drinking may result in sacking, repeated sackings, and then virtual unemployability. But it can also lead to more subtle and insidious processes: inefficiency, getting in people's way, leaving others to do a job, creating unpleasant situations, and so on. Medical practitioners may see this happening in their practices or in hospitals, and know how easily collusion and evasion develop.

There is reason to believe that unemployment may lead to increased drinking, since it is accompanied by five factors that are associated in employed people with a high risk of heavy alcohol consumption: easy availability of alcohol; freedom from supervision; very high (redundancy) pay or very low income; strains, stresses and hazards; and preselection of high-risk individuals. However, there is little evidence to show that unemployment in itself leads to heavy drinking. Although a number of population surveys have indicated that there is a higher prevalence of heavy drinking among the unemployed, it is not possible to tell from the data whether heavy drinking is the result of becoming unemployed, or vice versa *(105,106)*.

The bulk of alcohol-related crime consists of petty offences committed by people caught up in a way of life characterized by social instability — people who are unskilled, who do not stay for long in one job, who are homeless and often itinerant between cities, and who are in many ways socially and personally handicapped. Studies of prisoners in England & Wales have suggested that between one half and two thirds of men and about 15% of women have a serious problem related to alcohol *(107)*.

A recent investigation in England revealed that 64% of those arrested had been drinking in the four hours prior to their arrest *(108)*. Between the hours of 10 p.m. and 2 a.m. some 93% of all arrested persons were intoxicated. Alcohol use in the previous four hours was associated with 78% of all assaults, 80% of breaches of the peace and 88% of arrests for criminal damage. In some cases intoxication may predispose people to break the law. Others report drinking before committing a crime so as to reduce anxiety.

The association of drinking with hooliganism has led to controls on the availability of alcohol at football matches in some countries. Loss of self-control may be related to some sexual crimes, including rape, and is associated with some crimes of violence. In about half of all murder cases the assailant was intoxicated at the time, and often the victim would have been drinking *(109)*.

The final point about drinking and crime concerns convictions for drunkenness. The rates for this type of conviction run parallel to changes in per capita alcohol consumption. A high proportion of convictions for drunkenness are recurrent convictions for the same individual.

Rates for drinking-and-driving offences also run parallel to changes in per capita alcohol consumption. (Of course, conviction rates are related to the degree of police activity as well as to the amount of drinking.) A mass of evidence has now accumulated that demonstrates the relationship between drinking-and-driving and accidents. The most conclusive comes from a survey conducted by the Police Department in Grand Rapids, Michigan, USA *(110)*. For every person who had an accident the blood alcohol level was assessed. Control information was obtained by stopping motorists at the same accident point and checking their blood alcohol levels. At 80 mg per 100 ml of blood alcohol, the accident risk was twice the level of those who were sober; at 150 mg per 100 ml the risk was 10 times and at 200 mg per 100 ml it was 20 times the normal.

Furthermore, most traffic accidents in which alcohol plays a part seem to occur in regular heavy drinkers rather than among lighter drinkers who simply happen to have been caught. A recent study among motorists arrested for drinking-and-driving in the Tyneside region of Scotland demonstrated that although there was a relationship between blood alcohol concentrations and accidents among young drivers, the relationship did not hold for older drivers *(111)*. There was, however, a relationship between blood γ-glutaryltranspeptidase levels and accidents in older offenders. Young drivers are generally inexperienced with both alcohol and driving, and the acute effects of alcohol may make the dominant contribution to accident risk in this age group. Older drivers may be more experienced and relatively more resistant to the acute effects of alcohol. Accidents in the older group could therefore be due to a combination of acute and chronic deterioration in driving skills, the latter resulting from alcohol-induced neuropsychological deficiencies.

The strong association between raised γ-glutaryltranspeptidase activity and accidents in drivers over 30 years of age indicates that a large proportion of these accidents may be accounted for by heavy drinkers. Particularly disturbing in this study was the high prevalence of raised enzyme activity found among drivers of heavy goods and public service vehicles.

Countries such as Finland that carry out random breath-testing have demonstrated that it is an effective deterrent, leading to large reductions in both the number of drunken drivers on the road and deaths from road traffic accidents *(112)*.

Psychological damage
Psychological damage merges imperceptibly into social and physical damage and there are of course no hard and fast divisions between these three groups. For example, there is obvious overlap between social difficulties in the family, and psychological mood and the effects of conflict. The same is true of cognitive impairment and damage to the nervous system.

Most people are familiar with acute intoxication, and have experienced it to some degree at one time or another. Slurred speech and impairment of coordination, thinking and memory often occur. Ultimately, drowsiness results. Respiratory depression and inhalation of vomit can kill. Tolerance to some of these effects is acquired with regular heavy consumption, and whereas a blood-alcohol level of 150–200 mg per 100 ml may cause an inexperienced drinker to be obviously intoxicated, some regular heavy drinkers may appear superficially "normal" with a blood alcohol level of 500 mg per 100 ml.

One of the effects of intoxication is loss of judgement. Even though psychopharmacologically alcohol acts as a depressant, people paradoxically feel stimulated, at least after the first few drinks. This may mean, for example, that a person feels able to drive better, even though the evidence is that driving accidents are more likely even at blood-alcohol levels below 80 mg per 100 ml. Similarly, many people who feel they need to project a more attractive and confident appearance think that having a few drinks helps them to do so. In fact, the reverse is often the case. People become boring, loquacious, irritable and sometimes violent.

Alcohol is sometimes used to relieve unpleasant feelings such as anxiety and depression. There is, however, evidence that persistent heavy drinking, rather than relieving these feelings, actually exacerbates them. An individual may find his or her depression or anxiety getting worse, and mistakenly drink more in an effort to cope with these feelings. This is an example of one of many vicious circles that can be set up by drinking to excess. It is often very difficult to determine to what extent anxiety and depression are the result of heavy alcohol consumption, and to what extent they are the cause of it.

For someone who is beginning to become aware that his or her drinking is causing harm, or for someone who is well aware of that harm but finds it difficult to control the drinking, another set of vicious circles arises due to associated feelings of conflict and guilt. When people feel guilty about their behaviour, they have a tendency to minimize its extent and the harm it is causing, to try to cover it up, to become more secretive about it, and to rationalize it. It is important to appreciate that when this occurs, it is a natural psychological response to the real distress which the patient is feeling. Some of the more extreme forms of behaviour that are occasionally found in association with excessive drinking, such as abnormal jealousy and impulsive risk-taking, may have the same origins.

A feeling of low self-esteem is universal among people who are drinking to excess. The effect of this, combined with increased anxiety and depression as well as conflict and guilt, undoubtedly contributes to the very high rate of attempted and successful suicide among heavy drinkers.

Quite apart from impairment of judgement during acute intoxication and the effects of persistent drinking on mood and behaviour just discussed, regular heavy drinking may produce more general cognitive impairment. "Morning-after" amnesia quite often accompanies very heavy bouts of drinking, but frequent and more lasting periods of amnesia give warning of a serious risk of progressive damage, as well as being alarming for the person who has them.

As many as half of all the superficially normal heavy drinkers in alcohol treatment units manifest a detectable impairment of cognition and memory when subjected to formal psychological testing (113). They recover these faculties partly if they abstain, but age and the length of the drinking history increase the degree of impairment. It is not yet clear whether sustained but only moderate drinking leads to mental impairment (114).

Anyone could in certain circumstances become tolerant to alcohol and experience withdrawal symptoms. The main factor is exposure to prolonged heavy doses of alcohol. Although delirium tremens can develop within a few days of alcohol being withdrawn or severely cut down, and fits occur after 24 hours of abstention, primary care physicians are much more likely to be faced with the early features of tolerance and withdrawal. These occur typically on waking after the previous night's drinking, and extend from slight anxiety, anorexia and nausea to severe retching and vomiting. There may be tremor, ranging from slight hand movements to shaking of the whole body, and sweatiness, ranging from mild moistness of the hands to soaking sweats that drench the bedclothes.

Use of other drugs
Particularly in people with easy access to other drugs, such as doctors, nurses and pharmacists, the heavy use of alcohol may be linked with overuse of tranquillizers, hypnotics and other drugs. Young people perhaps alternate between using amphetamines, cannabis or other fashionable and illegal drugs and heavy drinking. There is a marked association between heavy smoking with its attendant risks and drug and alcohol consumption.

Physical damage
Both acute intoxication and regular heavy drinking can have an adverse effect on physical health. Alcohol can damage nearly every organ and system of the body, and lead to premature death.

Alcohol provides 7.1 kilocalories per gram, so that a standard bottle of 70° proof spirit provides 1500 calories. It contributes substantially to the obesity of many moderate drinkers, but on the other hand prolonged heavy drinking may lead to malnutrition and reduced levels of circulating vitamins. Although poor dietary intake and poor socioeconomic background contribute to malnutrition, this is not the whole story. In a study of middle-aged, middle-class heavy drinkers in the United Kingdom, 29% showed evidence of malnutrition (115). There was no correlation between nutritional status, dietary intake and the severity of liver disease.

54

Impaired intestinal absorption occurs in heavy drinkers, and may be due to impaired intestinal function and inhibited biliary and pancreatic secretions. Such malnutrition contributes to many of the alcohol-related diseases.

Alcohol has a direct toxic effect on developing erythroblasts, leading to macrocytosis which can occur in up to 90% of very heavy drinkers (116). It also inhibits the production and function of white blood cells, contributing to an increased susceptibility to infection. Megaloblastic anaemia occurs only in those who have nutritional folate deficiency, and so is more common in people with a poor dietary intake and in those who drink wines and spirits. Both contain negligible amounts of folic acid as compared to beer, which contains 100 micrograms per litre.

Alcohol exacerbates heartburn, and is a common cause of gastritis. Although cirrhotic patients have a high frequency of peptic ulcer, it does not seem that the ulceration is actually caused by the alcohol intake. Moreover, there is no noticeable difference in the healing and relapse rates of the ulcers, whether the patient continues to drink or stops (117).

A heavy alcohol consumption increases the risk of cancer of the mouth (excluding the lip) and pharynx threefold, of the larynx fourfold, of the oesophagus twofold (118). This effect seems to be irrespective of the type of beverage and is independent of cigarette smoking. However, alcohol and smoking together multiply the risk: the relative risk for cancer of the oesophagus may be 150 times higher in a heavy drinker and heavy smoker. A heavy alcohol intake may also be associated with an increased incidence of cancer of the colon and rectum (119).

Although they are rare, cancers associated with alcohol are among the few types of cancer whose rates have been increasing in recent years in countries where alcohol consumption has also gone up (120).

There is also an association between alcohol consumption and both acute and chronic pancreatitis (121).

Excess alcohol consumption can lead to a wide range of liver diseases, from fatty liver, hepatitis and cirrhosis to primary hepato-cellular carcinoma. Mortality from cirrhosis is 10 times the average in heavy drinkers. Liver injury is unrelated to the type of beverage consumed; it is related only to its alcohol content. Women develop liver disease after drinking less and for a shorter time than men, and at present seem to have relatively more severe liver disease (122).

The steady daily drinker is more at risk than the "spree" drinker whose total alcohol intake may be no less. In two studies on defined populations in France, the relative risk of cirrhosis compared to an alcohol consumption of 0–2.5 units per day was 6 times greater at 5–8 units per day and 14 times greater at 8–10 units per day (123). Above this level, though, the cirrhosis rate appears to be independent of both the duration of heavy alcohol consumption and the amount of alcohol consumed.

55

Only about 10–15% of heavy drinkers develop cirrhosis. Liver function tests show severe impairment in 25% of heavy drinkers and a lesser degree of impairment in 50%. It seems that alcohol sets the scene for potential liver damage but that an additional factor is needed to actually induce cirrhosis. Either genetic influences or possibly the hepatitis B virus may determine susceptibility. As many as 11% of individuals with cirrhosis will develop liver cancer as a late complication *(118)*.

There is a linear relationship between alcohol consumption and blood pressure that is independent of age, weight and cigarette smoking *(124)*. The Kaiser-Permanente study demonstrated a relationship between alcohol consumption and systolic and diastolic blood pressure (Fig. 9) *(84,125)*. The Yugoslavian study of cardiovascular disease demonstrated that high alcohol consumption was associated with a twofold increase in the risk of death from stroke, an effect accounted for by raised blood pressure *(76)*. Big alcoholic "binges" may also lead to strokes *(126)*.

Attenders at alcohol treatment clinics have raised blood pressure, which falls when they abstain *(127)*. It has been shown that one third of attenders at hypertension clinics may be heavy drinkers, and it has been suggested that for one in three of these heavy drinkers alcohol could be the direct cause of their hypertension *(124)*. Excess alcohol intake is probably the most common identifiable cause of raised blood pressure.

Alcohol directly causes a congestive type of cardiomyopathy that can develop in well nourished men after they consume half a bottle of whisky a day for several months *(128)*. Even in heavy drinkers without symptoms, echocardiographic studies frequently demonstrate an increase in left ventricular mass. "Binge" drinking may lead to cardiac arrhythmias, particularly atrial fibrillation *(129)*.

There seems to be reasonably clear evidence that moderate amounts of alcohol protect against cardiovascular disease *(83,130)* (Fig. 10).

Some 9% of heavy drinkers admitted to alcohol treatment units have chronic organic brain syndromes *(113)*. The frequency of these syndromes is higher in women (21%) than in men (7%), and increases with age and the duration of drinking in both sexes.

Only one quarter of those with clinical evidence of brain damage have the classic Wernicke-Korsakoff's syndrome. The remainder probably have brain damage due to cortical atrophy. In men without clinical evidence of brain damage, CAT brain scans demonstrate an increased sulcal width in about 40%. This is associated with a loss of white matter from the cerebral hemispheres *(131)*. Significant changes can occur in heavy drinkers below 40 years of age, but surprisingly the duration of drinking and the quantity of alcohol consumed do not correlate significantly with the severity of radiological abnormalities.

Both a peripheral neuropathy and acute and chronic forms of myopathy occur in heavy drinkers. The myopathy can occur independently

56

Fig. 9. Blood pressure related to alcohol consumption

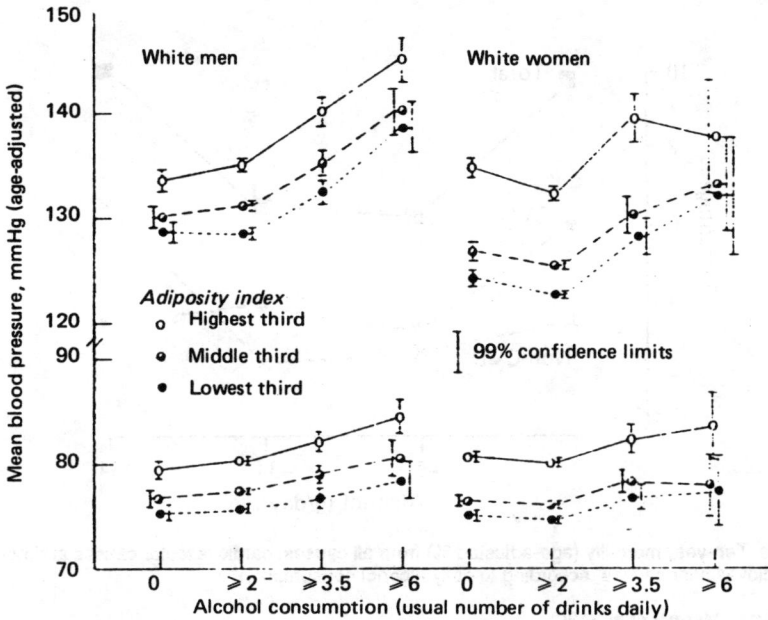

White men

White women

Adiposity index
o Highest third
ø Middle third
• Lowest third

I 99% confidence limits

Mean blood pressure, mmHg (age-adjusted)

Alcohol consumption (usual number of drinks daily)

Source: Alcohol — reducing the harm (42).

of the neuropathy *(132)*. Electrophysiological evidence for neuropathy and myopathy may be found in up to one half of heavy drinkers attending alcohol treatment units.

It is well known that intoxication leads to impotence and impairment of sexual performance. Regular heavy drinking also impairs sexual function. Loss of libido, reduced sexual activity, gynaecomastia and testicular atrophy occur in about one half of heavy drinkers attending alcohol treatment units, irrespective of liver damage *(133)*. Even moderate amounts of alcohol consumption (6 units per day) are related to impotence and male infertility. Of 90 men attending a male infertility clinic in the United Kingdom, 40% were thought to have low sperm counts as a result of drinking 4–6 units of alcohol a day.

Many heavily drinking women complain of sexual difficulty such as reduced responsiveness, and of menstrual problems such as cycle irregularities, menorrhagia and amenorrhoea.

Alcohol may damage the pancreas, and a comparison between countries reveals a relationship between alcohol consumption and diabetes mellitus *(134)*. On an individual level, a high alcohol consumption is a risk factor for the development of diabetic retinopathy *(135)*.

57

Fig. 10. Alcohol and mortality (The Whitehall Study)

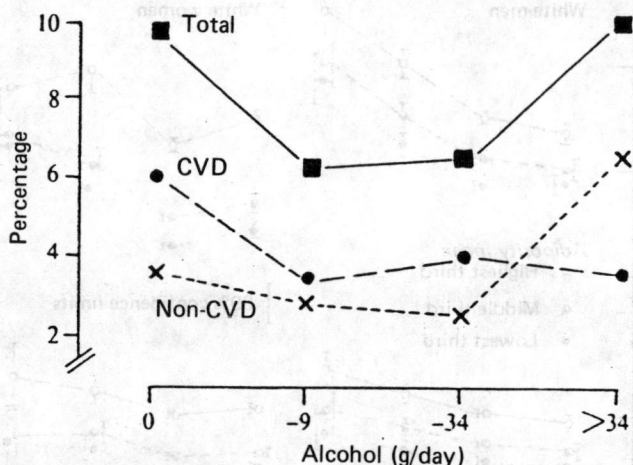

Note. Ten-year mortality (age-adjusted %) from all causes, cardiovascular causes and non-cardiovascular causes, according to daily alcohol consumption.

Source: Marmot et al. *(130)*.

Few babies are born to very heavily drinking women. The main reason is that liver damage leads to anovulation and amenorrhoea *(133)*. Heavy alcohol intake in pregnancy is associated with a combination of fetal abnormalities, including dysfunction of the central nervous system, growth deficiency and abnormal facial characteristics *(136)*. These abnormalities may occur in about one third of children born to mothers drinking the equivalent of half a bottle of whisky a day, although affected children show considerable individual variation in the extent and severity of damage.

Moderate drinking during pregnancy is associated with an increased risk of spontaneous abortion, stillbirth, congenital malformation and growth retardation *(136,137)*. In a recent study in the United States, which was controlled for the effects of cigarette smoking, the relative risks of spontaneous abortion during the second trimester of pregnancy were 0.13, 1.98 and 3.53 for women taking less than 1, 1–2, and more than 3 units of alcohol daily, compared to non-drinkers *(138)*. In a United Kingdom study, there was an association between alcohol consumption of more than 12 units per week and an increased risk of low birth weight *(139)*. The results of these and other studies led the US Surgeon General to advise pregnant women to abstain completely from alcohol *(140)*.

However, other factors are also associated with birth abnormalities, some of them apparently more important than alcohol. These include maternal age, social class, tobacco, use of illegal and prescribed drugs, obstetric history and diet. Recent evidence does not suggest that normal consumption, for example one or two units once or twice a week, has any harmful effect on fetal development *(141)*.

There is considerable evidence that even moderate doses of alcohol may be a risk factor for breast cancer in women *(142,143)*. In a follow-up study of women attending alcohol treatment units in the United Kingdom, mortality from breast cancer was twice the national rate *(82)*.

The relationship between drinking and road traffic accidents has already been discussed, but alcohol is also a significant cause of other accidents. Excluding traffic accidents, nearly two thirds of men admitted with serious injuries to accident and emergency facilities in the United Kingdom have blood-alcohol levels indicative of their having drunk 12 or more units *(144)*. About one third of home accidents are alcohol-related, and heavy drinkers have a work accident rate three times higher than normal *(145)*. In the United Kingdom, alcohol is the most common single factor in death by drowning; in 1983 drinking was implicated in 25% of such deaths. Also in the United Kingdom, alcohol consumption has been noted to be a factor in over two fifths of deaths from falls, and in two fifths of deaths from fires *(146)*.

Alcohol interacts with a wide variety of drugs. It prolongs the effects of tranquillizers (particularly benzodiazepines) and of antipsychotic and antidepressant drugs. Drugs such as barbiturates, beta-blockers and antihistamines impair psychomotor performance when taken with even a little alcohol. In the regular heavy drinker, as a result of enzyme induction, the metabolism of anticonvulsants, benzodiazepines, warfarin and sulfonylureas is speeded up. If liver disease develops, then the metabolism of many drugs will again become slowed.

Individual Risk and Level of Consumption

Many individuals are concerned to know their personal risk at different levels of alcohol consumption. Unfortunately there is a wide variety of opinion about safe or sensible levels of drinking.

A number of authors have studied the relationship between consumption and damage *(147,148)*. While it is clear that heavy drinkers have higher rates of morbidity and mortality than light drinkers, in many studies heavy consumption has not been defined. It has either been implied *a priori*, for example in studies of alcohol-clinic attenders, or defined loosely without reference to any minimum volume of intake. One exception to this is the study by Péquinot et al. already referred to *(123)*. This study showed that men who consumed between 28 and 42 units of alcohol a week had a risk of developing cirrhosis six times that of men with a weekly consumption of less than 14 units, and this risk increased to 14 times for men drinking between 42 and 56 units a week. Another exception is the United Kingdom civil servants study, which demonstrated an increased mortality for men consuming more than 30 units of alcohol a week *(130)*.

Of course the averages of alcohol consumption referred to in most studies are simply the total volume of alcohol consumed over a given period of time, divided by the number of days or weeks involved. They do not take into account differences in patterns of drinking, although the pattern appears to be irrelevant to most alcohol-related conditions, except in so far as it affects the total amount of alcohol consumed. (Where it is evidently highly relevant, on the other hand, is in acute problems such as accidents.) Nor does the type of beverage seem to make much difference, although folate deficiency is associated with wine and spirits consumption, cancer of the oesophagus is possibly associated with spirits consumption, and colorectal cancer possibly with beer.

Many studies fail to take into account individual susceptibility to alcohol. A number of investigations have suggested that women may be more susceptible to the toxic effects of alcohol than men. Following a standard oral dose of alcohol, their blood-alcohol values are significantly higher than men's. Tissue ethanol concentrations are also correspondingly higher in women, and it is reasonable to suppose that over a period of time this might result in earlier or more severe tissue damage. Women who drink heavily develop fatty liver, hepatitis, cirrhosis of the liver, obesity, anaemia, malnutrition and gastrointestinal haemorrhage faster than men *(148)*. Alcohol influences women differently at different times of the menstrual cycle.

Alcohol may do disproportionate damage at the extremes of youth and old age, and ethnic origin may also be important in determining susceptibility. Provided these two caveats are borne in mind, Table 22 gives a reasonable guide to personal risk at different levels of consumption.

Table 22. Guide to risk at different levels of alcohol consumption

Risk	Weekly consumption	
	Men	Women
Low	Less than 20 units	Less than 15 units
Moderate or intermediate	21–50 units	16–35 units
High	50 units or more	35 units or more

Population-Attributable Risk

It is now clear that although heavy drinkers have a lot of alcohol-related problems, their contribution to the total number of such problems in any country is small *(149)*. The majority of alcohol-related problems are attributable to the relatively large number of light and moderate drinkers, although only a small proportion of them have alcohol-related problems. This is similar to what happens in the case of high blood pressure or high serum cholesterol, and is illustrated in Table 23 (see overleaf).

Implications for primary health care physicians

Clearly, alcohol causes widespread problems that need to be recognized as alcohol-related and dealt with accordingly within the primary health care services; this is particularly important in the management of chronic conditions such as diabetes and raised blood pressure.

It is difficult to obtain figures for the contribution heavy drinking makes to the workload of the primary health care physician. The General Household Survey in the United Kingdom has demonstrated that, compared to light drinkers, heavy drinkers have more health problems and consult their general practitioners twice as often *(151)*. In the second national study of morbidity in primary health care in the United Kingdom, 0.9 per 1000 patients consulted for alcoholism and drug dependency. The rate was 1.1 per 1000 patients for those aged 25–44 years, and 1.7 per 1000 for those 45–64 years of age, out of an overall consultation rate per 1000 population for these age groups of 4.5 and 6.5, respectively *(152)*. Wilkins *(153)* estimated a prevalence rate of 11 per 1000 population aged 15–65 for present "alcoholics" in his practice.

Table 23. Alcohol consumption and mortality: the effect of reducing alcohol consumption on death rates in middle age

Units of alcohol per week	Percentage of population in this band [a]	Ten-year death rate per 10 000 population [b]	Death rate if everyone reduced consumption to next lower band	Number of lives saved per 10 000 population in ten-year period if everyone reduced consumption to next lower band
Band 1: 1–10	60	600	600	—
Band 2: 11–35	30	900	600	90
Band 3: 36 +	10	1200	900	30

[a] Wilson (21).
[b] Klatsky et al. (150).

4

Resources

In most countries there is little prospect of a significant increase in the resources allocated to health services, despite the fact that the demand will grow with an aging population and as new diagnostic and therapeutic techniques are developed. The biggest dilemma facing politicians and managers seems to be the competition between two "boxes" or areas of care: hospital care and community care. However, this two-box concept is inaccurate. The hospital, no matter how specialized, is a community service. Hospital staff may focus on the individual rather than the whole population, but hospitals serve the community, and hospital and community services are not mutually exclusive but interdependent. And there are not two boxes of health care but four *(154)* (Fig. 11). Hospital and community care provide less care than the informal care provided by family, friends and volunteers and self-care, which are the other two boxes.

Health care planning (which is at present dominated by hospital planning) and mortality statistics must be reoriented simply because hospital and mortality data are the most easily accessible sources of data. These vitally important components of planning should be complemented by information on the health needs of the whole community, not just those who die or those who use the hospitals.

The World Health Organization's principles of primary health care planning provide a useful checklist for this type of planning. Primary health care planning embraces hospital planning and is based on the following four principles.

1. The needs of the whole population should be considered and not just the needs of those in contact with the health service.

2. Resources should be used effectively and efficiently.

3. Health service planning should be interrelated with the planning of other services.

Fig. 11. The four-box system of health care

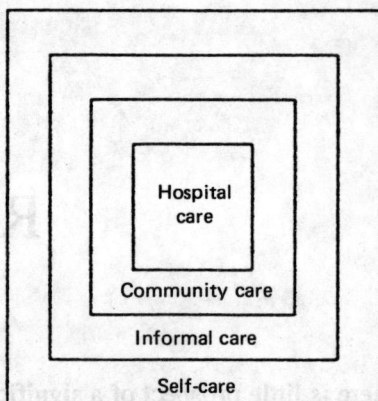

```
┌─────────────────────────────────────┐
│  ┌───────────────────────────────┐  │
│  │  ┌─────────────────────────┐  │  │
│  │  │    ┌─────────────┐      │  │  │
│  │  │    │  Hospital   │      │  │  │
│  │  │    │    care     │      │  │  │
│  │  │    └─────────────┘      │  │  │
│  │  │   Community care        │  │  │
│  │  └─────────────────────────┘  │  │
│  │        Informal care          │  │
│  └───────────────────────────────┘  │
│              Self-care               │
└─────────────────────────────────────┘
```

Source: Gray *(154)*.

4. Users of the service should be involved at all stages of planning and development.

Some rational planning work has been done on the provision of specialist alcohol services *(155)*. There are four planning steps. The first is to determine the population to be served by geographic area and size. The basic approach is to define service areas according to existing planning jurisdictions, and to determine the population of these areas from existing census data.

The second step is to estimate the number of problem drinkers and alcohol-dependent drinkers in each population unit. Using, for example, alcohol sales data and per capita consumption data, it is possible to estimate the distribution of alcohol consumption in the various planning jurisdictions. For each planning area an estimate is made of the number of people drinking at various levels of risk. The risk categories correspond to the average number of standard drinks consumed per day. Using this method, the number of people consuming at a particular level is used as an approximate measure of the number of people at various points along the continuum of problem severity.

The third step in planning is to estimate the number of individuals out of those counted in step two who should be treated in a given year. At this stage an estimate is made of the proportion of the in-need population who should be planned for on an annual basis. This population can be referred to as the target or the demand population. There is general agreement that the percentage of problem drinkers who are currently seeking or who have recently sought treatment is quite low.

The fourth step is to estimate the number of individuals out of those counted in step three who will require service from each component of the treatment system. For specialized services it is possible to define different service categories (Table 24) and then, using various published sources of data, to estimate the proportions of individuals who should be allocated to the various treatment categories. Using this model it is possible to define the need for different services at each of the planning locations. An inventory of existing services can be drawn up *(156)* and the need can then be balanced with the actual provision. Oversupply of services can be reduced in favour of unmet need.

Table 24. Examples of service categories

Category	Description
Assessment/referral	Systematic procedures for the identification of a client's major strengths and problem areas culminating in a treatment plan and referral(s) for assistance.
Detoxification	Services provided to clients who are intoxicated or in withdrawal from alcohol and/or other drugs. These may be provided under medical supervision or in a non-medical detoxification centre.
Case management	The process of monitoring, tracking and providing support to a client throughout the course of his/her treatment and after.
Outpatient treatment	Treatment provided on a nonresidential basis, usually in regularly scheduled sessions (e.g. 1–2 hours per week).
Day treatment	Intensive, structured nonresidential treatment, typically provided five days per week (e.g. 3–4 hours per day).
Short-term residential treatment	Intensive, structured treatment provided for a period of time while the client resides in-house. The length of stay is typically less than 30 days.
Long-term residential treatment	Treatment and/or rehabilitation services provided for a period of time typically longer than 30 days. These programmes include recovery homes, half-way houses, and three-quarter-way houses.
Aftercare	Resources or services that provide continuing encouragement and additional services as needed, following a client's completion of a treatment plan.

Source: Rush *(155)*.

Community Involvement and Health Promotion

It is important for local communities to be involved in planning and developing strategies for the prevention and management of alcohol problems *(157,158)*. The City of Oxford in the United Kingdom is a good example of this. The City Council has a Healthy City strategy with 25 target "health areas" corresponding to the WHO targets for health for all. One of these health areas is the prevention of alcohol problems. The City Council and the Department of Public Health carried out an audit of the City Council departments (Table 25) to find out what they were doing in the way of health promotion. The departments then listed what else they might do in the future, and each department is now filling in a matrix (Fig. 12) which sets targets, proposes strategies, lists programme objectives and specifies outcome indicators.

Another example of community work is the development of policies for managing alcohol use in municipally owned recreational facilities *(159–161)*. For example, Thunder Bay in the Province of Ontario, Canada adopted a policy of regulating the use of alcohol so that consumption was not permitted in some facilities, was limited to special occasions requiring a special permit in others, and was fully licensed in a third group. The policy was decided on with the support of the local community. An evaluation showed that after its implementation there was a shift in behaviour and attitudes on the part of the public in favour of the policy.

Some researchers have looked at how licensed traders can be involved in the promotion of sensible drinking *(162–165)*. Server liability is a rapidly changing area of legal policy: citizens' groups and some government agencies think it an appropriate response to the drinking-and-driving problem *(166–170)*. Both legislators and the courts have reacted to this, so that commercial servers of alcohol now find themselves in greater jeopardy of being sued because of the actions of their under-age and intoxicated patrons. Unfortunately, though, there has not yet been enough research done to help licencees fulfil their perceived responsibility to the public. However, server liability laws do have the potential to bring about a dramatic change in retailing practices so that they take health and safety into account.

When community resources are used for the prevention and management of alcohol problems, it is important to begin with community surveys of the drinking habits of the local population *(171)*, their beliefs about alcohol *(172)* and their beliefs about health promotion *(173)*. The surveys should be planned and executed with the involvement of the community. They not only provide information, but also get the community involved as a resource, and have another spin-off because members of the community may themselves identify areas of need in terms of prevention or resource provision *(3,174–176)*.

66

**Table 25. City of Oxford
Council Departments**

Environmental Health Department
  Housing section
  Health promotion and liaison section
  Food section
  Noise pollution section
  Pollution section
  Occupational health section

Personnel Department

Department of the Chief Executives

Department of City Secretaries

Department of Engineers and Recreation
  City Engineer's section
  Recreation section

Department of Housing

Department of Planning, Estates and Architecture

Of course, a wide range of agencies are jointly responsible for the community response to alcohol-related problems.

Self-Help and Self-Care

The most common kind of health care is self-care, but its importance is often underestimated by professionals, who overlook the fact that even a person receiving the maximum of support from community services is usually alone for perhaps 22 hours a day. Self-care is not an alternative to professional care, since it includes the use of professional services. Indeed, the promotion of self-care increases certain demands on community and hospital services, although it reduces others. Primary health care physicians are already trying to influence people's decisions about referral from self- and informal care to community care, by trying to discourage those who repeatedly seek help for conditions they could safely and effectively manage themselves. There is now increasing evidence that self-care is effective in cutting down on drinking. Vaillant's study, for example, showed that apart from the emergence of medical problems made obviously worse by drinking, other factors that

67

Fig. 12. City of Oxford target health area matrix

Health area	Target population	Activity	Present services provision	Department target	Strategy to achieve targets			Programme objectives	Standards	Outcome measures
					Structural change	Knowledge change	Behavioural change			
Environmental health										
Housing										
City Engineer and Director of Recreation										
Planning, estates and architecture										
Personnel										
Chief Executives										
City Secretaries										
Treasury										

helped Boston men to abstain were the discovery of substitutes for alcohol (not all of them innocuous) and the formation of new and rewarding relationships *(49)*.

Heather *(177,178)* has also reported on the use of self-help manuals by problem drinkers. Some 785 people responded to a newspaper advertisement offering free help to cut down on drinking, and were sent alternately either a self-help manual based on behavioural principles or a general information and advice booklet. Of the total, 247 (31.3%) returned assessment questionnaires or agreed to be interviewed by telephone; and of these, 132 (53%) were successfully contacted at six-month follow-up. Those lost to follow-up were significantly more stable socially than those recontacted. Among the latter, there had been a significantly greater reduction in the previous weeks' alcohol consumption in the group who had received the manual (40%) than in the control group (25%) and there had also been significantly greater improvements in physical health and in the degree of social interaction.

Informal Care

The three main sources of informal care are the family, friends and voluntary organizations. Many studies have stressed the importance of family support. Saunders & Kershaw *(179)* confirmed this once again when they studied people who considered that they had had a drinking problem in the past, but not any longer. When these people were asked for reasons by far the most common answer was marriage; others included obtaining work or now having better working conditions.

While undoubtedly many family members can be seen as victims of the stress resulting from one person's drinking problem, a systems view of families is probably more helpful in both understanding the family's role and helping them to help the drinker *(48)*. With the systems view, the family are treated as an indivisible system of people playing independent roles. The use of alcohol in the family is purposive, adaptive and meaningful. In assessing the way the family is working, one considers what functions excessive drinking may be serving for the family as a whole, not just for the individual identified as a problem drinker; it could well be a signal of a family problem at one level or another. This kind of understanding of family dynamics may increase our ability to help the family in both the prevention and management of alcohol problems. So, while planning for service provision, we recognize the importance of family members in enabling the heavy drinker to drink less (see also p. 127) and provide support also for them.

More attention should be paid to the high levels of stress experienced by families with a drinking problem, and also to the family members' role in the continuation or successful resolution of the problem. The partner of an identified problem drinker should always be involved in management if possible, and there should be a comprehensive counselling and advice service for partners alone in cases where the drinker is unavailable for treatment.

Alcoholics Anonymous is a classic example of a voluntary organization that encourages the exchange of information and advice between sufferers from the same complaint. It is a fellowship of men and women who believe that the only way to cope with their alcohol problem is to give up drinking completely. Activities are usually concentrated at the local group level. The only requirement for membership is a desire to stop drinking, and a determination to stay stopped. The mutual aid process of Alcoholics Anonymous demands openness. Members have to be open with each other about their past, their activities, their relationships and their emotions. Alcoholics Anonymous also operates an open membership policy, in which the characteristics that are sometimes used to distinguish people such as age, sex and religion are ignored, while the one thing that members share — their alcohol problem— is emphasized. Also, members of Alcoholics Anonymous have to be open to the possibility of change. It is an essential part of the mutual aid process that members help each other to modify their self-perception, their network of friends and relationships, and even the style and content of their everyday life.

However, while for many people Alcoholics Anonymous is a supportive self-help group, for many others it is not the answer. It is unfortunate that the organization has done little in the way of research into its own effectiveness.

Primary Health Care

In recent years there has been a shift towards providing minimum treatment for problem drinkers (180) and basing this minimum treatment in primary health care (181). The nature of primary health care services and the way in which they relate to specialist services varies considerably throughout the European countries.

There are four typical approaches to organizing primary medical services in the industrialized countries of Europe. In some, there is a relatively uncoordinated system of general practitioners and specialists working independently, either singly or in group practice; here, the patient essentially makes the first choice about whom to consult. In others, and particularly in the socialist countries, most of the population are served by polyclinics. In densely populated areas these can be very large, providing facilities for up to 50 physicians, the majority of them being specialists. In sparsely populated rural areas the polyclinics are smaller and general practitioners usually work alone. In some countries, such as the United Kingdom, a general practitioner is responsible for a group of patients who have chosen him or her as their primary care physician. The general practitioner is then responsible for referring any patients for whom a specialist opinion is sought. In the Scandinavian system the focal point for the provision of care is not a specific named practitioner but a health centre run by the local administrative unit. The area of responsibility here is defined not so much by individual choice as by administrative boundaries. The personnel working in the health centre are salaried employees, and again specialists may be found working in this setting.

In some countries, therefore, access to specialist services is only through the primary health care physician, while in others the client may choose to make direct contact with the specialist who may be working in the front line of health care.

The prevention and management of alcohol problems is well within the role of primary health care. Since alcohol problems are associated with significant morbidity and mortality, there is no doubt about their importance to a primary health care system. In addition, the deleterious effects of excessive drinking on the family are well recognized. Primary health care offers a low cost intervention that does not require a group of alcohol specialists but relies principally on the skills of individuals who are already in post and accessible to the population they serve. Finally, the primary health care setting has the quality of reproducibility to the extent that it consists of a network of similar services, and a pilot scheme that has proved effective in one part can readily be replicated in other parts.

Primary health care is also a beneficial setting because there is evidence that excessive drinkers suffer more ill health than others and therefore make more than average use of health facilities. Primary health care physicians and nurses are usually accessible to the community and have an established credibility that enhances any advice they may give. The primary care setting also avoids the problems of stigma and labelling, which often arise when a patient is treated by specialist alcohol services, and it is the ideal setting for health promotion work (182,183).

Despite these advantages, there are a number of barriers to early intervention in the primary care setting (184–187). Primary health care physicians and nurses may overlook alcohol's contribution to a patient's presenting problem. Another barrier is the health worker's pessimism about the value of any intervention, which coupled with the known unpopularity of alcoholic patients suggests that a certain amount of resistance may have to be overcome before primary health care workers feel comfortable with the responsibility for this task.

Many primary health care staff feel inadequately trained to deal with alcohol problems. A preliminary task in designing alcohol programmes for the primary health care setting would therefore be to organize training

71

in the recognition of problems, probably involving the use of screening instruments, and training in giving clear advice appropriate to a particular patient's pattern of harmful drinking *(186)*. The studies reviewed in this book show that simple intervention strategies can be effective. This should convince primary health care workers that there is a valuable and effective part for them to play in minimizing the damage done by alcohol. The new role need not be onerous or time consuming. It does not call for the acquisition of specialist skills, and by reducing the likelihood of further alcohol-related health damage it should save time and resources.

Community-based preventive medical departments
Some health care systems offer population-based preventive services. For example in Malmö, a southern Swedish city of about 230 000 inhabitants, an Institute of Preventive Medicine in the Medical Department of Malmö General Hospital has been in operation since 1975. The programme is directed against the major medical health risks and complications of middle age such as cardiovascular diseases and alcohol consumption. The Department is equipped for both screening and intervention, which are oriented mainly to the needs of the individual. To date, 35 000 middle-aged residents of Malmö have been invited to come to the Institute; of these 25 000, or just over 70%, have attended. Risk factors are classified in terms of markedly abnormal values, leading to referral to the Medical Department; intervention levels, taken care of in the outpatient clinics; and borderline levels, checked by repeat tests by the nurses over 1–2 years *(188)*.

Occupational health
Alcohol-related problems affecting workers have become a serious concern in many countries *(189)*. There is general recognition of their serious consequences, not only for the workers themselves but also for families and colleagues, employers and society at large. At the same time it has become increasingly apparent that the workplace is an appropriate and advantageous setting for dealing with these problems. There is a growing interest in educational and assistance programmes started jointly or separately by employers and trade unions, or by public authorities and nongovernmental organizations.

There are a number of good reasons for supporting programmes at the workplace.

1. The majority of problem drinkers are part of the workforce.

2. For most people, work is the most highly structured part of their daily life. The signs and symptoms of a developing alcohol problem are constant, predictable and identifiable at the workplace. A fall-off in work performance is easily recognized, and problems tend to be harder to hide.

3. The workplace provides a unique opportunity for support and assistance from co-workers, who often notice things going wrong long before management and supervisors do.

4. The possibility of being fired can be used as an important motivating factor for change.

5. It is more cost-effective for employers to encourage problem drinkers to go for treatment than to sustain the cost of continuing poor performance, premature retirement or accidents.

6. The chances of recovery are much lower for problem drinkers who are out of work. They are also likely to become a bigger burden on society.

7. The workplace is a good place for health education.

Community alcohol teams
The United Kingdom now has a number of services based on the community alcohol team models *(190–192)*, which arose from the Maudsley Alcohol Pilot Project. The community alcohol teams were based in the community rather than in hospitals, their purpose was to help primary health care workers respond to a variety of problems associated with alcohol, and their members came from different professions including psychiatry, nursing, social work and psychology.

The function of the community alcohol team was to support groups of primary care workers while simultaneously providing them with information, training them, and helping them gain experience in working with drinkers. The teams did this in two ways: through training courses and by a consultation service. It was recognized that merely telling primary health care workers the size of the alcohol problem and that it was their responsibility to respond to it was not enough. The team was based on the concept that primary health care workers must be given active help; that their rights and responsibilities must be clarified; and that they must be given information about specific problems involved in actual cases. They must also be given concrete proposals as to how to translate this information into a therapeutic response, and most important of all they must be supported and supervised when carrying it out.

Evaluation of the community alcohol teams has shown, however, that the concept is difficult to put into practice *(191)*. The teams have in fact developed into additional tiers of specialist services, bringing these services into the community rather than helping to create a truly community-based response at the primary health care level.

General Hospitals

General hospitals are an ideal setting for making therapeutic contact with problem drinkers *(193)*. Heavy drinking is linked to many physical diseases, and studies of the drinking habits of general hospital patients have revealed that the likelihood of being admitted to a general hospital for liver disease, myocardial infarction and upper gastrointestinal tract diseases begins to increase in men who drink more than 30 grams of alcohol per day. Attenders at hospital injury departments also have high rates of positive blood-alcohol tests and other markers of regular alcohol intake. A number of studies in the United Kingdom have shown that in general hospitals that serve mainly urban areas something between 15% and 30% of male admissions and between 8% and 15% of female admissions are of problem drinkers.

Screening procedures and interventions for problem drinkers can be devised, therefore, in the general hospital. A number of interventions are possible, using general hospital staff, specially trained staff or voluntary lay counsellors. Nevertheless, there are certain difficulties. First, in general hospital wards problem drinkers have often not yet begun to see their problem as alcohol-related, or to accept that it would be advisable for them to alter their drinking habits. The second difficulty is that there is a lack of interest among general nursing and medical staff, as well as pessimism about treating patients with alcohol problems. The training of these staff in management of the problem drinker should therefore aim to dispel negative stereotypes, to improve detection rates, to inculcate simple counselling and communication skills, and to enable staff to provide advice to the heavy drinker.

An alternative approach might be to use a specially designated and trained staff member to counsel problem drinkers. Voluntary lay counsellors could also be invited to counsel problem drinkers in hospitals. Their efficacy would clearly be greatest if their approach to the patient were given the full weight of the physician's authority, and if the physician had already begun a dialogue with patients about their drinking.

The casualty department should ideally have a worker attached who can take referrals from busy casualty staff. In city centre departments, a social worker in the casualty department can play a valuable role by assessing individuals with alcohol problems and either using the opportunity to open a dialogue with them or making a referral.

In all instances follow-up is important. Often the primary care physician will be the appropriate person to do this.

Community-Based Programmes

During the last 10 years there has been a shift towards providing services through community programmes rather than hospital-based care, with an associated change in the types of treatment offered. Hospitals operate mainly according to a medico-organic model that focuses on the medical

74

or psychiatric management of alcohol-related problems, whereas community-based services adopt a psychosocial approach to treatment based mainly on individual and group counselling, although other psychological techniques are also employed.

The main aim of a recent randomized control trial was to compare the services offered by a community-based day centre with the conventional inpatient and outpatient management provided by a district general hospital. No differences in outcome were found between the two patient groups in terms of psychosocial and biochemical indices, but patients in the community-based group had a greater reduction in average daily alcohol consumption at one-year follow-up than those in the hospital-based group.

Obviously both the general hospital and community-based centres are potential sources of treatment for problem drinkers, but the community-based centre is cheaper and more accessible.

Specialist Treatment Services

Most countries have a wide range of both outpatient and inpatient specialist services but there have been changes of direction here too in recent years, partly because of their relative effectiveness (49,194–198), but also because it is now recognized that specialist services can be offered to only a minority of those with alcohol-related problems.

It is now known that, in hospital, anti-alcoholism programmes of a few weeks to a few months are no more successful than brief periods of hospitalization lasting only a few days. Day-treatment programmes have been found to be equal or superior to hospitalization, at one half to one third of the cost. Outpatient programmes are comparable in terms of results with inpatient programmes, and permit considerable savings per patient. A growing body of evidence now suggests that if patients could be clinically matched to a range of treatment alternatives, much higher overall improvement rates would be observed (198).

The result of all these findings has been that specialist services now provide outpatient, day patient and community care rather than intensive inpatient care. In fact their role has changed, so that in future specialized staff will actually be supporting primary health care. During a transitional period the specialist services will need to be strengthened and specialists helped to convert to more consultative and educational activities as trainers of primary health workers (192).

Detoxification Services

Detoxification is an approach that has been proposed particularly for single homeless drinkers. These are only a small minority among problem drinkers, although they are often the most visible and easily identified. However, attempts to find the best type of programme for this group have been unrewarding. Detoxification services have not been shown to be effective in terms of either rehabilitation or decriminalization *(199,200)*. The term "detoxification service" in fact covers a variety of quite different things in different countries, including hospital inpatient units, inpatient units experimenting with support in place of medication, non-hospital residential projects, hospital outpatient services, and detoxification at home. In the research literature this diversity has rarely been acknowledged, and in the present state of knowledge overall conclusions about the effectiveness of detoxification services are quite unwarranted.

An alternative and more realistic idea may be individual monitoring of service users. This approach, similar to the single-case-design approach of psychology or the case-study approach of the social services, should help to track an individual's path through various agencies and forms of accommodation, including the detoxification services. It could lead to better collaboration and integration between those agencies that recruit or refer people for detoxification, those that actually carry it out, and those that provide further treatment or rehabilitation.

5

Promoting health and preventing damage

Chapter 4 summarized the data linking the consumption of alcohol with alcohol-related damage. The public health implications of this link are obvious: prevention is everybody's business and everybody's responsibility. It is clear that there would be a very significant drop in the overall level of alcohol-related damage if alcohol consumption could be reduced. But how could such a reduction be brought about? Many international committees, governmental and professional, have pored over this problem *(201–212)*. (National policy issues will not be dealt with in detail here, as they are covered in a previous WHO publication *(213)*.)

National Influences on Consumption

On an individual basis genetics, personality, attitudes, beliefs, religion, culture, age, sex, occupation, social class, experience, exposure and area of residence all determine how much people drink, how they drink, and how and whether they are damaged by their drinking. Many factors determine how much a *society* drinks, but four of them — all controllable — emerge as the most important: price, availability as determined by licensing laws, advertising and health education.

Price and fiscal policy
The economic components of prevention policies have been fully reviewed elsewhere *(214)*. Briefly, there is an inverse relationship between the real price of alcoholic beverages on the one hand, and the level of consumption per head and most indices of alcohol-related harm on the other. Fig. 13 shows the price relative to income per litre of absolute alcohol consumed in the United Kingdom during the period 1949–1979, the percentage of consumer spending on alcoholic drink, and litres of alcohol consumed. As the relative price of alcohol fell — by over 50% — alcohol consumption increased accordingly.

Fig. 13. The relative price of alcohol in Britain, 1949–1979

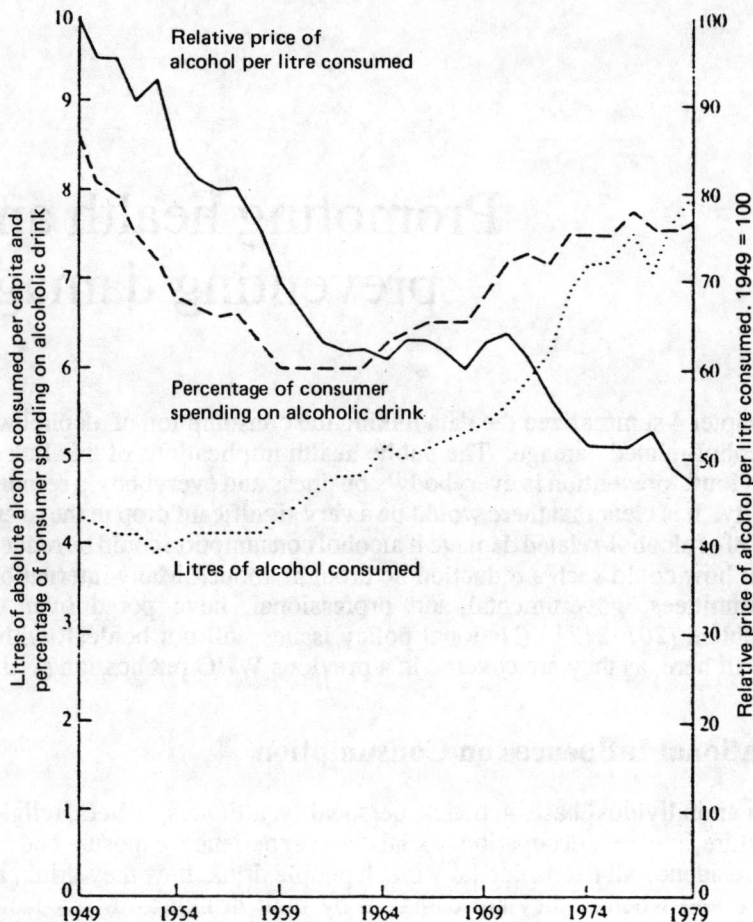

Source: Alcohol — reducing the harm (42).

Table 26 shows the strikingly close correlation between consumption, the relative price of alcohol, and deaths from cirrhosis in Ontario from 1928 to 1967. Popham et al. *(65)* studied all the data available in various jurisdictions and concluded that "almost universally relative price was found to be very closely associated with indices of consumption and alcoholism". International comparisons of relative price and consumption provide further evidence of this.

Using time-series regression analysis to investigate the relationship between income and price on the one hand, and consumption on the other, it is possible to quantify the income and price elasticities of demand for

Table 26. Consumption of alcohol, relative price of alcohol, and
deaths from liver cirrhosis, Ontario, 1928–1967

Year	Per capita alcohol consumption in litres of absolute alcohol	Relative price	Deaths from liver cirrhosis per 100 000 population over age 20
1928	2.81	0.102	4.4
1931	2.64	0.112	4.0
1934	2.09	0.137	4.2
1937	3.36	0.086	4.5
1940	3.64	0.074	5.0
1943	4.91	0.064	4.8
1946	5.82	0.069	5.4
1949	7.18	0.058	7.2
1952	7.32	0.051	7.7
1955	7.55	0.047	8.8
1958	7.96	0.043	11.0
1961	8.14	0.043	11.6
1964	8.73	0.039	11.9
1967	8.91	0.035	13.2

Source: Popham et al. (65).

alcoholic products (215,216). The price elasticity of demand is a measure
of the responsiveness of the demand for a product when its price changes
by a small amount. The income elasticity of demand is a measure of the
change in the demand for a product when the income of consumers
increases by a small amount (217).

A report by the United Kingdom Treasury suggests that for a 1% rise
in its relative price, consumer demand for beer might be expected to fall
by about 0.25%, for spirits by 1.5%, and for wine by 1% (218). However,
a 1% rise in real incomes might be expected to increase consumer demand
for beer by about 0.75%, for spirits by 2.25%, and for wine by 2.5%. This
suggests that over the years the consumption of beer, the predominant
drink in the United Kingdom, has been less sensitive to changes in price
and income than consumption of wine and spirits, and that the consumption of alcoholic drinks in general is less sensitive to rises in prices than
to rises in disposable income. Fig. 13 also shows that the percentage of
consumer spending on alcoholic drinks in the United Kingdom increased
from 6% in 1960 to just under 8% in 1979.

It has been suggested that high alcohol taxes are regressive in that
they tend to lead to a less acceptable distribution of income after tax. In
so far as the poor spend a higher proportion of their income on alcohol
than the rich, they also pay a disproportionate share of the tax on alcohol.
However, the evidence for this is not strong. There are differences

between alcoholic beverages with regard to consumption patterns. In Britain, beer figures more predominantly in the budgets of low rather than high income groups, but spirits and wine are luxuries in the sense that high income groups spend relatively more on them than low income groups, and also spend a more proportionate share of any increase in income on them.

The freedom of many European countries to fix taxation levels for alcoholic drinks is circumscribed by the Treaty of Rome. The European Community is seeking to create a common market in alcoholic drinks by removing internal barriers to trade, and also wishes to harmonize tax levels so that alcohol products are treated equally by the tax systems of all member countries. The effect that the resulting price falls and increases in consumption will have on the number of alcohol-related problems is obvious. Successful harmonization and competition policies in the European Community will oblige such countries as the United Kingdom to reduce their relatively high levels of wine taxation. It is estimated that such a change would lead to an increase in alcohol consumption in the United Kingdom of 30%.

Availability and licensing laws

A country's licensing laws determine the terms and conditions under which alcoholic drinks are made available to the public. In some countries the issuing of licences is a local matter, with the licensing laws providing the legal framework within which local licensing magistrates must work. Although the total number of retail or supply outlets increased by 29% between 1945 and 1980 in the United Kingdom, the increase in relation to population size has been only 8% (219). Nevertheless, many people believe that the increased availability of alcohol in, for example, supermarkets has contributed to the rise in alcohol-related problems, particularly among women.

There are in fact many plausible reasons why an increase in the number of licensed premises might stimulate consumption: easier access, for example, and an increase in point-of-sale marketing efforts such as window stickers and displays inside supermarkets. Econometric studies done in the United Kingdom suggest that a 1% reduction in the number of licensed premises might reduce the total amount of alcohol consumed by around 2% (220).

Licensing hours are another way of controlling availability. However, studies on the effects of licensing laws in general are sparse, and many national committees have made their recommendations for licensing changes without having much hard evidence to support them. It has been suggested that ''civilized drinking'' should be encouraged, meaning the kind of drinking that goes on in a French cafe with soft drinks, non-alcoholic beverages and food available, and with long opening hours and a family atmosphere rather than, for example, the sort of drinking done in a Scottish pub where furniture, politeness and women are all at a minimum. This is a subjective rather than an objective judgement, however. Although Scotland has a high rate of problems related to intoxication, France has a death rate from cirrhosis ten times higher. "Tavern diversification" was tried in Ontario in 1978, but did not lead to any slowing of the increase in consumption over the following five years as compared with Manitoba, where no changes were made.

There is some historical evidence of the influence of licensing, however. Licensing laws were first introduced in Britain in 1914, in an attempt to discourage drunkenness among munitions workers, and alcohol consumption fell dramatically over the next few years. In Finland, on the other hand, a new law introduced in 1969 and intended to relax controls led to a 22% increase in the number of shops selling alcohol, a 32% increase in the number of restaurants with a full licence, extended opening hours, lower age limits on sales, and 3000 more cafes and 17 000 more shops selling beer. The result was that consumption suddenly shot up by 47% (11).

Scotland relaxed its licensing laws in December 1976. Since then public bars have been allowed to remain open for an extra half hour in the evenings, whereas before they were obliged to close at 10 p.m., and subsequently public houses were permitted to open on Sundays, previously a privilege enjoyed only by hotel bars and licensed clubs. Some all-day licences — that is, regular extensions of permitted hours — have also been issued by the licensing courts, which were themselves introduced during 1977.

The impact of the Scottish changes has been the subject of much debate. Trends in alcohol-related morbidity and mortality from 1970 to 1982 compared with trends in England & Wales show no specific changes related to the 1976 relaxation, but appear to be a continuation of those evident between 1970 and 1976 (221) (Fig. 14). However, officially recorded rates for drunkenness have declined more in Scotland than they have in England & Wales (Fig. 15). This could be due to many factors but is probably attributable more to changes in police policy than to a more relaxed or civilized style of drinking (22,222).

In the United Kingdom, however, it does seem that the licensing laws have done much to keep the country near the bottom of the international league tables for consumption and alcohol-related harm (Fig. 16) (201).

Advertising
Research evidence is equivocal concerning the effect of advertising on the total amount of alcohol consumed. The alcohol and alcohol-advertising industries maintain that advertising affects brand choice, rather than the overall level of alcohol consumption. Nevertheless, there is evidence that changes in beverage preferences tend to be additive rather than substitutive, suggesting that brand or beverage switching may result

81

Fig. 14. Total alcohol-related mortality in Scotland and in England & Wales, 1970–1982

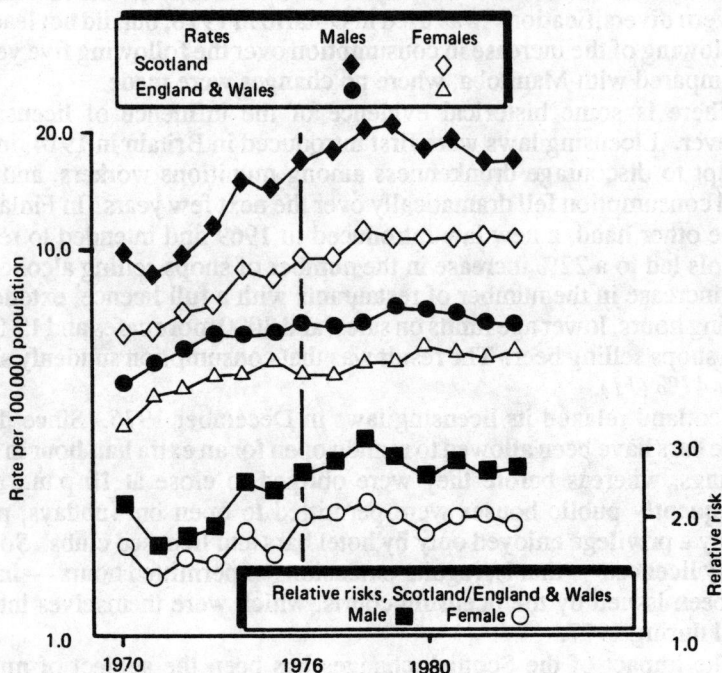

Source: Duffy & Plant (221).

in greater total alcohol consumption (223). The results of research conflict, but generally they show a low elasticity of demand with regard to advertising (224,225). Any attempt to control advertising expenditure would, it seems, have little effect on the demand for beer, wine or spirits but could, if successful, reduce the companies' costs and enable them to cut prices.

An alternative would be to impose a specific advertising levy on alcoholic drinks, thus increasing the cost of advertising to the companies. To maintain former advertising levels they would have to finance this additional cost, which in turn would increase their overall costs, narrow their profit margins and possibly lead to price increases, with associated potential effects on consumption. Other alternatives would be to persuade alcohol producers to reduce their levels of advertising voluntarily or in certain circumstances ban it altogether. British Columbia introduced a total ban on alcohol advertising in 1972 (226) and Manitoba

Fig. 15. Convictions for drunkenness and drink-driving in Scotland and in England & Wales, 1970–1982

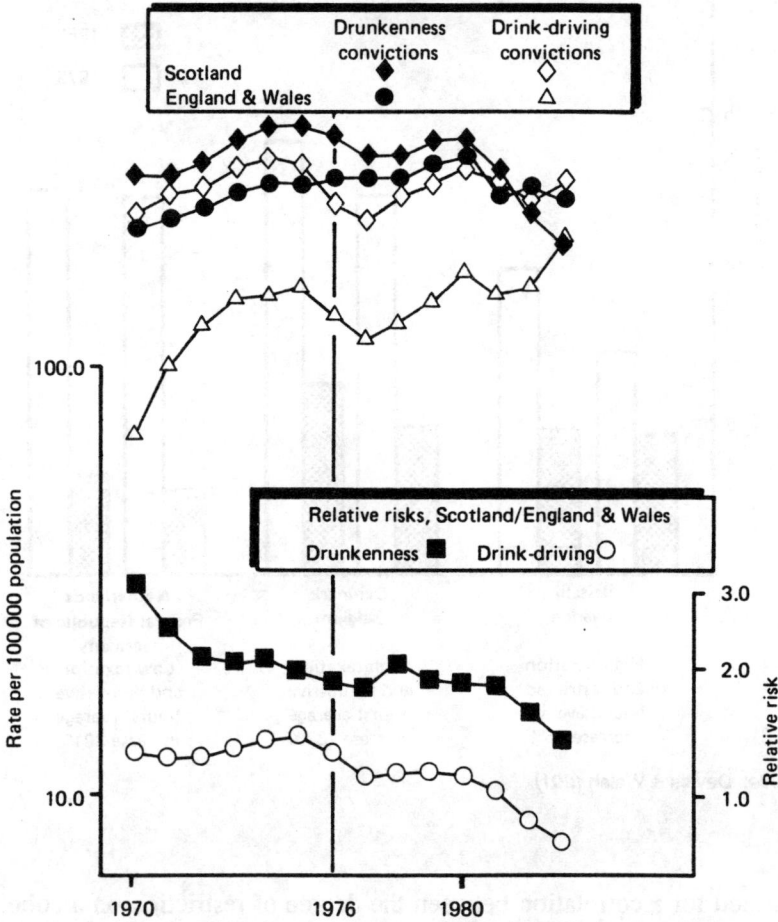

Source: Duffy & Plant (221).

banned beer advertising in 1974 (227); in neither case was there a dramatic change in consumption. It is difficult to interpret these results, however, since the two populations concerned were still exposed to the media of both the United States and other Canadian states to which the bans did not apply, and neither the communities nor the mass media supported the bans.

There is not much evidence either as to the effectiveness of restrictions on the style and content of advertising. Ogborne & Smart (227)

Fig. 16. Alcohol consumption trends in the six main beer-drinking countries of North-west Europe, 1950–1979

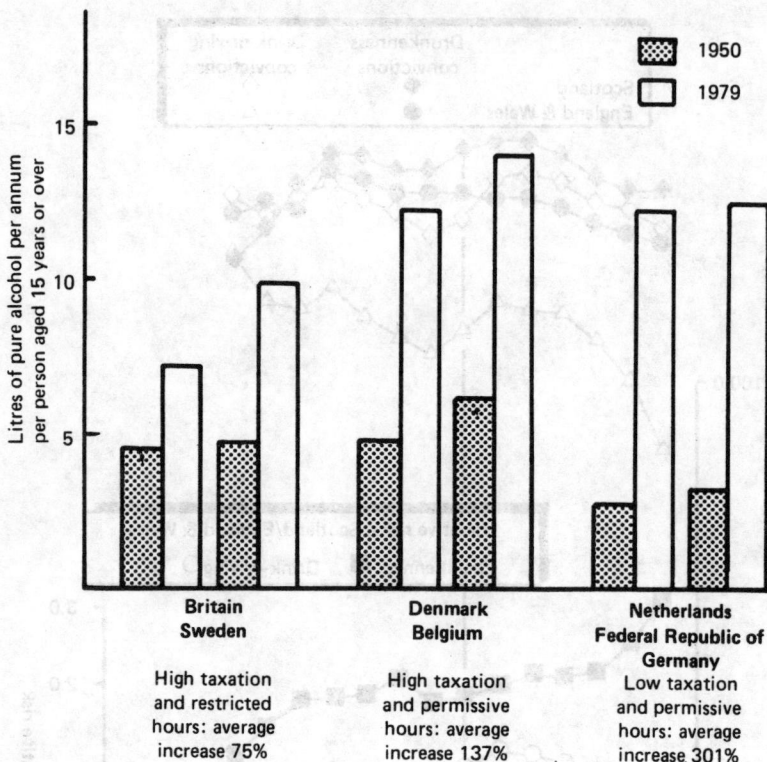

Legend:
- 1950 (shaded)
- 1979 (open)

Y-axis: Litres of pure alcohol per annum per person aged 15 years or over

Britain Sweden	Denmark Belgium	Netherlands Federal Republic of Germany
High taxation and restricted hours: average increase 75%	High taxation and permissive hours: average increase 137%	Low taxation and permissive hours: average increase 301%

Source: Davies & Walsh (201).

searched for a correlation between the degree of restriction on alcohol advertising in the 51 United States and consumption, but could find none. Nevertheless, a number of countries believe the content of alcohol advertising *is* important. Any unpalatable ideas, images and messages may be rejected by the majority, but they can be absorbed by certain potentially vulnerable groups such as the young, and it is believed that they can promote or reinforce harmful patterns of consumption.

As a result of concern about the impact of the media, some countries have introduced regulatory controls of advertising content. In the United Kingdom, for example, alcohol advertising is dealt with specifically in both the Independent Broadcasting Authority (IBA) Code of Advertising Standards and Practice, which governs all advertising in the broadcast media, and the Advertising Standards Authority (ASA) British Code of

Advertising Practice (BCAP), which regulates all advertising in non-broadcast media. Among other things the IBA Code forbids: the portrayal in alcohol advertisements of any personality commanding the loyalty of the young; any suggestion that drinking is essential to social success; the portrayal of "round" buying; the association of alcohol with driving or using potentially dangerous machinery; and the portrayal of regular or solitary drinking.

Health education
The mass media are one of the most seductive and compelling elements in everyday life, and are credited by some with a power and influence that are perhaps exaggerated. Consequently everyone from politician to potato grower uses the media as a way of exerting influence. The alcohol health educator is no exception (228); so far, however, there is little evidence that health education about alcohol problems has been successful in reducing them. In 1976 the Scottish Health Education Unit mounted a national campaign on alcohol problems (229). The campaign used television and press advertising, and its main aim was to encourage people with problems to come forward for treatment. Although many did, the general level of public knowledge was not significantly increased, and patterns of alcohol consumption did not change. A campaign in the north-east of England showed that specific media campaigns for alcohol education are very expensive and only modestly successful in imparting knowledge (230). It does appear that the more culturally and class sensitive the material the more effective the message, but this rules out transferring regionally produced material to national networks, and in practice makes effective material very costly.

The main aim of publicity should be to encourage the mass media to put the prevention of alcohol-related problems on their agenda and to get accurate information, whether about facts or about concepts, over to the public.

There is an EC proposal to label all alcoholic drinks with their alcohol content by volume. Potentially this could be helpful in informing consumers of the quantity consumed, since at present beers may vary from 1% to 8%, table wines from 8% to 16%, and spirits from 37% to 45% alcohol by volume. In addition cider, thought by many to be low in alcohol content, may actually exceed 20% alcohol by volume. However they are measured, it is important for the consumer to understand that a drink is a drink whatever the beverage and contains about 10 g of alcohol in most European countries.

National policy-making
The drinks industry, governments and health lobbies all participate in determining national preventive policy. The industry is immense, rich and powerful on both national and international levels (217,231). In many countries the markets for beer, wines and spirits are dominated by

85

large multinational firms *(232–234)*, which are often not single-product alcohol firms but also major producers of tobacco and other goods. There are extensive links between the different components of the markets involved in alcohol production, distribution and retailing. Moreover, in many countries the trades concerned have expanded very rapidly; in certain parts of various countries, the majority of the population in some towns and villages are directly dependent on alcohol for a living.

The power of the alcohol trades is mediated through industrial lobbies working at local and national levels, with representatives in governments and elsewhere. In addition, alcoholic drinks account for a high proportion of industrial activity, contributing to exports and raising a considerable proportion of government revenues. Poised between the industry and the public health lobbies, a government may often find itself facing in many different directions. In the United Kingdom, for example, 18 different government departments have some interest in alcohol (Table 27). These include the Department of Health, concerned with the health effects of alcohol abuse; the Home Office, which controls licensing; the police, who deal with drunkenness and with crime and traffic accidents due to alcohol; the Department of Transport, also concerned with road accidents; the Department of Employment, concerned with industrial accidents, absenteeism and their effects on output; the Treasury and Customs and Excise, concerned with tax and revenue collection; the Ministry of Agriculture, Fisheries and Food, which sponsors the alcohol industry; the Ministry of Defence, concerned with the effects of excessive drinking in the armed forces; and the Department of the Environment, which is concerned with football hooliganism and with sports sponsorship by the alcohol industry. Until recently there has clearly been too little coordination between the many government departments and agencies that have a hand in alcohol-related matters. A number of governments, including now those of both France and the United Kingdom, have set up interdepartmental ministerial committees to coordinate the government's response to alcohol problems.

Local Action

Apart from the national strategies discussed so far, there are local initiatives that primary health care physicians can take to promote the health of their own communities. Many of these will call upon the wealth of largely untapped preventive resources in every community, which the primary health care services can help to mobilize *(236)*.

Local alcohol policies
Local communities, health authorities and councils can develop their own prevention policies *(236)*, possibly as part of the WHO health for all and Healthy Cities initiatives (see p. 66). Such policies can include a

86

Table 27. Government departments in the United Kingdom with an interest in alcohol

Government department	Interest
Department of Health and Social Security	Trends in the effects of alcohol consumption. Health and social service provision for victims of alcohol misuse. Health education on alcohol. Sponsoring research into alcohol abuse and related problems.
Ministry of Agriculture, Fisheries and Food	Sponsorship of the alcohol industry, including distribution and retailing. International aspects (trade) that bear on the wellbeing of industry. Regulation of drinks for purity, etc. Nutritional aspects of alcohol consumption.
Home Office	Licensing law. Offences of drunkenness. Other criminal offences associated with consumption of alcohol and treatment of offenders with alcohol problems. Police interest in drink-related road accidents. Broadcast advertising of alcoholic drinks, in the context of the Home Office sponsorship responsibilities for broadcasting.
Law Commission Office	Function of JPs in licensing laws.
Department of Transport	Road accidents and related legislation (Great Britain, in association with the Scottish Office).
Department of the Environment	Football hooliganism, as affected by alcohol (with the Home Office). Sponsorship of sport by the alcohol industry.
Customs and Excise	Duties on alcoholic drinks, including international negotiations.
Treasury	Fiscal policy. Prices. Balance of payments for trade in alcohol. Economic significance of the alcohol industry. Public expenditure effects of alcohol abuse.
Department of Trade	Prices. Competition and pricing policy as it bears on the alcohol industry, including distribution and retailing. Policy on container sizes and metrication. Consumers' interest in advertising and promotion. International trade in alcoholic drinks. Press and cinema film industries. Alcohol consumption in the Merchant Navy and the civil aviation industry. Tourism.
Department of Employment	Effect of alcohol abuse on accidents, absenteeism and productivity.
Department of Education and Science	Health education in schools. Effect of alcohol on young people in education.
Civil Service Department	Effect of alcohol abuse on the efficiency and conduct of the civil service.
Ministry of Defence	Policies affecting the control of alcohol in the Armed Services and the treatment of its misuse.
Scottish Office	
Welsh Office	
Northern Ireland Departments	

Source: **Alcohol problems** *(235)*.

package of activities that help to reduce both consumption and related problems. In each local community there are institutions, organizations and key individuals whose work can be used to influence consumption.

The provision of information
Many local authorities, institutions and individuals are concerned in some way with alcohol problems but are not necessarily aware of the public health implications of their work. They include social workers, probation services, police, magistrates and licensing justices, and they all need to be provided with regular information on the extent of alcohol consumption and the size and nature of the alcohol-related problems in their communities.

Primary health care teams, with their local knowledge and close involvement with the community, are ideally placed to collect and monitor information on alcohol-related problems and bring it to the attention of the individual and of the bodies just mentioned. For example, they can collect information on alcohol-related home accidents for home safety committees, or on the extent of heavy drinking for licensing justices. They can also encourage employers to adopt alcohol-at-work policies.

Media support
The media are important where prevention is concerned for two reasons. First, people who work in the media are among the heaviest consumers of alcohol and form one of the occupational groups at greatest risk of alcohol-related damage; and second, the media have a responsibility to adopt a balanced perspective on matters of public and social significance. This is especially important when issues such as the revision of licensing laws or duties and taxes on alcohol are being debated. The fact that there are individual and community costs of alcohol, as well as benefits, is often neglected in media coverage of alcohol-related issues.

Advertising and sponsorship
There are at least three things that local groups can do about advertising and sponsorship. First, they can make complaints about advertisements that appear to be in breach of advertising codes and standards, if such exist. If they do not, complaints can still be made about advertisements that are unhelpful in terms of the prevention of either consumption or problems. Second, local groups can take action to control poster advertising. In most localities the majority of poster sites are owned by local government authorities, which are thus in a position to control a highly visible form of mass communication. Control may mean a complete ban on alcohol posters, limiting them to particular areas, or limiting their overall number. And third, local groups can oppose the involvement of alcohol companies in sports sponsorship.

Licensing
In those countries that have licensing arrangements, it is the central government's role to provide the legal framework within which local licensing magistrates must work. However, it is up to the magistrates themselves to issue licences for the sale and serving of alcoholic beverages and to determine the frequency, type and location of licensed establishments in a local area. In the United Kingdom, for example, licensing magistrates have absolute discretion over the granting of licences for the sale of drinks to be consumed on (or off) the premises and they have a right, confirmed in case law, to base their decisions on an estimate of local need.

At first sight, therefore, the licensing laws seem to be a powerful instrument of control over the availability and consumption of alcohol in a locality. However, there are a number of reasons why they do not have the impact that might be expected. By and large, licensing magistrates have no special knowledge or understanding of alcohol-related problems, and especially not of the relationship between availability and consumption. Any attempt they make to restrict outlets can be challenged on appeal by determined applicants, and moreover the right of magistrates to define local need is balanced by an obligation to consider every licensing application on its own particular merits. As a result, many licensing committees have been forced to adopt an implicitly liberal attitude towards licence applications. They leave it to the market to decide whether the locality needs another outlet, rather than basing need on a declared licensing policy, or taking into account the public health aspects of licensing.

Given that many local individuals and organizations have a legitimate interest in licensing decisions, and could make a worthwhile contribution to them, it is a good idea to set up local licensing forums where all concerned can meet to discuss the introduction and implementation of an overall licensing strategy, how to raise support for it, and what kinds of data should be available to magistrates when decisions are made either on general issues of need or more specific questions such as the connection between licensed premises and public disorder.

Safety promotion
Many local networks are interested in alcohol in so far as it affects home, water and road safety: occupational health and safety groups (including personnel officers, supervisors and managers), the medical profession, trade unions, employers' organizations and insurance companies. Other groups that contribute to the safety network include pedestrians' and cyclists' associations, road and highway engineers, local government surveyors, coroners (who have a statutory right to comment and advise on the circumstances and conditions surrounding fatalities), local government home safety committees, road safety departments, the fire service,

89

hospital accident and emergency departments, and many more, not forgetting anti-drinking-and-driving organizations such as Mothers Against Drinking and Driving in the United States.

Alcohol issues should be a routine topic for most of these local networks. For example, the subject of alcohol and work should always be part of the training curriculum for health and safety officers and personnel managers, and fire brigades should routinely record any involvement of alcohol in fires. At present, few local authority home safety committees know much about the connection between alcohol and domestic accidents, and only a minority of hospital accident and emergency departments routinely record whether or not alcohol was involved in an accident.

6

Screening, case identification and assessment

Population Screening

Screening is now done for many physical and psychological disorders and has become an accepted part of health care. Before it can be endorsed for a particular disorder, however, the minimum requirements are that there should be a significant benefit to health and wellbeing to be gained from it, and that screening should result in earlier detection and treatment of the condition than if the person screened had presented spontaneously *(237)*.

The main criteria for screening are as follows *(237)*.

1. The condition should be an important health problem.

2. There should be a recognizable latent or early symptomatic stage.

3. Treatment at the pre-symptomatic or early symptomatic stage should favourably influence the course of the condition and the prognosis, and should therefore be preferable to no treatment.

4. There should be agreement as to who is to be treated.

5. The treatment should be generally available.

6. There should be a suitable screening test for detecting the condition at the early symptomatic stage.

7. The cost of identifying, diagnosing and treating cases should be supportable within the budget for medical care as a whole.

Alcohol-related damage fulfils most of these criteria.

The practical value of a screening *instrument* is limited by the time, skill and resources needed to carry out the procedure. In one country manpower may be a limiting factor, in another skill and/or technology. Self-administered questionnaires are very practical, although there may be difficulties as regards repeatability and validity. Repeatability influences the extent to which a single item of measurement can be taken as a guide to action. Self-completed questionnaires are liable to within-subject variability only, so further measurements can be taken later and an average calculated. Validity can be assessed by comparing the screening-test results with the results of a reference test, usually a full clinical investigation. Two kinds of error may be revealed: false-positive and false-negative classifications. False-positive results can lead to needless alarm, whereas false-negatives may lead to some individuals not receiving treatment from which they would benefit. A specific test is one that yields few false-positive results, and a sensitive test is one with few false-negatives. Unfortunately, attempts to make a test more specific usually have the effect of making it less sensitive.

When a test is first applied it is not enough just to know its sensitivity and specificity: one must also know how likely it is that a person with a positive test has the condition being screened for, or in other words the predictive value of a positive test. This predictive value depends on the prevalence of the condition in the group under study. As prevalence increases from 0% to 100%, so too does a positive test's predictive value. Understanding of this point is of practical importance: new screening instruments are usually tested first in hospitals or clinics, where prevalence is high, but the decision to use them for population screening depends on their performance in areas of low prevalence.

Screening for Alcohol Consumption

If we accept that alcohol is a risk factor for ill health, then we must conclude that it is necessary to screen for it. This can be done by the use of self-administered questionnaires. Questionnaires are necessary because, on the whole, primary health care workers are not aware of the drinking habits of their patients *(238)*.

Quantity/frequency questionnaires

Quantity/frequency questionnaires have been used in many alcohol research studies *(239,240)* (Fig. 17). Typically, they contain questions on the usual frequency of drinking over a certain period of time (a week or a month), the type of drink taken, and the usual quantity of each drink consumed per day; from this it is possible to calculate such measures as the average weekly alcohol intake. However, the quantity/frequency questionnaire has not often been used as a screening instrument until quite recently. Barrison et al. *(241)* combined quantity/frequency questions with the four CAGE questions (p. 96) in a survey of patients admitted to a general hospital, and Wallace et al. *(242)* used a similar approach with primary health care patients.

Fig. 17. Quarterly frequency measure of alcohol consumption

IN THE LAST MONTH: have you had an alcoholic drink at all? YES NO

If YES: please answer A and B

A. About how often have you had any of the following types of drink over the last month?

Beer, lager, cider, etc.	not at all	less than once a week	1–2 times a week	3–4 times a week	5–6 times a week	every day
Wine, sherry, vermouth, etc.	not at all	less than once a week	1–2 times a week	3–4 times a week	5–6 times a week	every day
Gin, vodka, rum, brandy, whisky, etc.	not at all	less than once a week	1–2 times a week	3–4 times a week	5–6 times a week	every day

B. When you've had a drink over the last month how much of the following types of drink have you usually had a day (i.e. 24-hour period)?

Pints of beer, lager, cider, etc.	none	½–1	1–2	3	4–5	6–7	8 or more
Glasses of wine, sherry, vermouth, etc.	none	1–2	3–4	5–6	7–9	11–14	15 or more
Measures of spirits (gin, vodka, rum, brandy, whisky, etc.)	none	1–2	3–4	5–6	7–9	11–14	15 or more

93

Quantity/frequency questionnaires have high test/retest reliability and substantial validity when compared with drinking diaries. It is important to offer respondents the option of recording a high alcohol intake *(34)*.

Quantity/frequency questions on tobacco use, diet and exercise, for example, have also been used in other health-related questionnaires for purposes of health promotion.

Drinking diaries
Seven-day diaries have been used in community studies, either retrospectively or prospectively, to ascertain the distribution and amount of alcohol consumption *(21)* (Fig. 18). But again they have not often been used as a screening tool, being more time-consuming and complicated than a quantity/frequency questionnaire. However, the diary has been shown to give more accurate information about consumption, with an estimated reliability of at least 90%. The mean daily consumption reported in quantity/frequency questionnaires has on average been about 66% of that indicated by diaries *(244–246)*.

A number of researchers have investigated underrecording in completed questionnaires *(27,29,30,33)* and have found that the tendency to forget the amount consumed varies according to the drinking measure employed. For example, respondents tend to underestimate their frequency of drinking and overestimate the quantity consumed on a typical drinking occasion. Between 8% and 17% of drinking occasions may be forgotten. The longer the time period asked about, the greater the number of occasions forgotten.

Deliberate underreporting of consumption may occur because of the stigma associated with heavy drinking and its behavioural effects, but there have been few empirical investigations into the actual extent of underreporting. It does seem, however, that the *degree* of underreporting increases with amount consumed. One British survey, in which a standard lie-scale was incorporated in the questionnaire, revealed that dissimulation reduced total weekly alcohol consumption by between 46% and 65% *(247)*. There is some evidence that higher consumption levels are reported when contact with an interviewer is reduced or eliminated altogether. In both general population *(248)* and alcohol-dependent inpatient studies *(249)*, computerized interviewing techniques have been shown to result in increased self-reported consumption levels as compared to interviews by human beings.

Measurement of Psychosocial Consequences

The first screening instruments used to detect alcoholism derived from the work of Jellinek, who conducted a survey of members of Alcoholics Anonymous and identified a series of questions that most characterized

94

Fig. 18. Example of a drinking diary

Day	How much?	When, where, who with?	Standard drinks	Total
Monday	1 pint beer	At lunchtime, in pub with Bob	2	2
Tuesday	Nothing		0	0
Wednesday	½ pint beer, 2 large whiskies	On way home from work, in pub, alone / At home, watching TV, alone	1, 4	5
Thursday	Nothing		0	0
Friday	2 glasses of wine, 2 pints of strong lager	At lunchtime / In pub after work with Bob	2, 8	10
Saturday	2 pints of beer and 2 double whiskies	Saturday night, in pub with John and Carol	4, 4	8
Sunday	2 pints beer, 3 glasses of wine	Before lunch, in pub with John / with lunch	4, 3	7
			Total for the week	32

Source: That's the limit. London, Health Education Council, 1983.

the experience of alcohol problems in those subjects *(250)*. Screening itself actually became popular in the 1960s, and since then many different self-administered instruments have been introduced.

Michigan Alcoholism Screening Test (MAST)

This 25-item interview comprises questions relating to personal opinions on drinking, opinions of family and friends, problems arising from drinking, and some symptoms of alcohol dependence *(251,252)*. In a population of hospitalized American alcoholics, the MAST was found to have a sensitivity of 98% in detecting alcoholism. It has been used principally in the United States and the United Kingdom in clinic populations. Pokorny et al. *(253)* devised a shortened version of the brief MAST (S-MAST), using the 10 most discriminating items from the original (Fig. 19). The questions asked are direct and unequivocal in their focus on alcohol: they require the respondent to admit that drinking is a problem. Kaplan et al. *(254)* found that self-identified alcoholics scored much higher on this test than did non-self-identified alcoholics.

The limited usefulness of the MAST as an early detection instrument was suggested by the original work of Selzer *(251)*, who found that it gave a positive diagnosis in only 55% of persons convicted of drunkenness and disorderly behaviour, and in only 11% of motor vehicle drivers whose licences were under review because of an alcohol-related offence. In a community study, Saunders & Kershaw *(255)* found that the MAST correctly identified only 50% of heavy drinkers. Kristenson & Trell *(256)* modified MAST by using questions about attitudes and customs rather than serious symptoms, which they felt would be more acceptable to a population of apparently healthy Swedish men. This instrument (Mm-MAST) correctly identified 73% of known alcoholics in their general population sample.

MAST has been used as a screening test in a family practice in both the United Kingdom *(257)* and the United States *(258)*, although no information is given about reliability or validity. Gibbs *(259)* recently reviewed its validity as measured against other diagnostic criteria for alcoholism, and summarized the evidence of its reliability. Although he could find only 12 studies that gave reliable information, the results indicated that MAST agreed with other diagnostic procedures in about three out of four cases. Where inconsistencies did occur, MAST tended to overdiagnose alcoholism. Gibbs found that evidence regarding the reliability of MAST was scant, with little test/retest reliability data available. It did appear that the shortened versions of MAST were less reliable than the longer versions.

The CAGE instrument

This questionnaire consists of only four questions *(260)*.

    1.   Have you ever felt you ought to CUT DOWN on your drinking?

Fig. 19. The brief MAST (S-MAST)

Question	Circle correct answer	
1. Do you feel you are a normal drinker?	Yes (0)	No (2)
2. Do friends or relatives think you are a normal drinker?	Yes (0)	No (2)
3. Have you ever attended a meeting of Alcoholics Anonymous (AA)?	Yes (5)	No (0)
4. Have you ever lost friends or girlfriends/boyfriends because of drinking?	Yes (2)	No (0)
5. Have you ever got into trouble at work because of drinking?	Yes (2)	No (0)
6. Have you ever neglected your obligations, your family or your work for two or more days in a row because you were drinking?	Yes (2)	No (0)
7. After heavy drinking, have you ever had delirium tremens (DTs), severe shaking, heard voices or seen things that weren't there?	Yes (2)	No (0)
8. Have you ever gone to anyone for help about your drinking?	Yes (5)	No (0)
9. Have you ever been in a hospital because of drinking?	Yes (5)	No (0)
10. Have you ever been arrested for drunk driving or driving after drinking?	Yes (2)	No (0)

Source: Pokorny et al. *(253).*

2. Have people ANNOYED you by criticizing your drinking?

3. Have you ever felt bad or GUILTY about your drinking?

4. Have you ever had a drink first thing in the morning to steady your nerves or get rid of a hangover (an EYE-OPENER)?

Two or more positive replies are said to identify the problem drinker. In the original study of 366 American psychiatric patients, 81% of known alcoholics answered positively to two or more questions, compared to 11% of non-alcoholics. The CAGE questionnaire has been used in psychiatric clinic populations *(260)*, general hospital populations *(261)*, patients of family physicians *(242,262)* and communities *(255)*.

When responses to the MAST, case-note review, quantity of alcohol consumed and diagnosis according to DSM are used as a standard, in general hospital settings the CAGE questionnaire has been shown to have a sensitivity as high as 85% and a specificity as high as 89% *(261)*. Used in a community survey, CAGE appeared to be more sensitive than the shortened MAST *(255)*; nevertheless it failed to detect approximately half of the known active alcoholics and problem drinkers in the community. In one family practice setting, the CAGE questionnaire was modified from simple "yes/no" answers to four graded options, ranging from "very often" through "often" and "sometimes" to "never" *(242)*. Some 46% of men consuming more than 35 units of alcohol per week (one unit contains about 8 grams of absolute alcohol) and 44% of women consuming 21 units per week or more were positive on the modified CAGE questionnaire.

Spare Time Activities Questionnaire (STAQ)
This questionnaire was used in England in a primary health care setting by Wilkins *(263)*. Initially, he constructed an at-risk register based on some of the known predisposing factors leading to an increased risk of alcohol problems. The STAQ attempted to disguise its alcohol focus by also asking about recreational pursuits such as watching television and participating in sports. The STAQ questionnaire is longer than the other instruments described, requiring 7–8 minutes to complete by a heavy drinker. Wilkins reported a sensitivity of 77%. Saunders & Kershaw *(255)* used it in a modified form in their community survey, and found it had good agreement with the CAGE questionnaire but that its power to detect known alcoholics was not better, as it identified less than 50%.

Munich Alcoholism Test (MALT)
The Munich Alcoholism Test involves a combination of a clinical assessment performed by a physician and a questionnaire completed by the patient *(264)*. The doctor assesses the level of the patient's consumption and indicates clinical findings. The questions asked are similar to those found in the MAST. An evaluation of this instrument demonstrated high validity and reliability, and there were no false-positives.

98

LeGo grid
LeGo *(265)* developed a diagnostic procedure based on physical stigmata associated with excessive alcohol consumption. The assessment consists of physical signs (appearance of skin, conjunctivae and tongue, and tremor of lips, tongue and hands) and of assessments of subjective complaints (liver volume and consistency, blood pressure and weight).

Validation of the grid demonstrated no correlation between LeGo ratings (controlled for age) and alcohol dependence ratings. There was, however, correlation with withdrawal symptoms, and with γ-glutaryl-transpeptidase (GGT) and serum aspartate aminotransferase levels *(266)*. The grid reflects the physical consequences of long-standing drinking, rather than drinking-associated dependence or psychological harm.

Mixed consumption/psychosocial consequences scales
A number of the scales referred to have been used in combination with measurements of alcohol consumption. For example, the CAGE questionnaire has been used with consumption measurements in both general hospital *(241)* and primary care settings *(242)*.

A questionnaire combining items on consumption with the four CAGE questions was used to detect abnormal drinking among 520 patients under the care of all the specialist departments of a general hospital in London *(241)*. Altogether, 108 of them were identified as meeting the criteria for excessive drinking on the basis of their replies to the questions on how much they drank. A total of 33 people answered "yes" to two or more of the CAGE questions, and all but five of these were identified as excessive drinkers on the basis of their admitted consumption levels. Thus 28 abnormal drinkers were detected by both methods; 22 of these were not only aware of having a drink problem as shown by a positive score on the CAGE, but were in fact admitted with a disorder that resulted from excessive drinking. The failure of the remaining 80 heavy drinkers to answer positively on the CAGE suggested that they either had no problems related to their drinking or were largely unaware of or unconcerned about any such problems.

The modified CAGE questionnaire and a quantity/frequency estimate of consumption were administered to 62 000 people registered with primary health care practices in the United Kingdom *(242)*. Positive responses to the CAGE questionnaire were obtained from 10.8% of men and 5.3% of women. Of the 1945 heavily drinking men (those consuming more than 35 units of alcohol per week) 46% expressed concern about their drinking by a positive CAGE response, as did 44% of the 989 heavily drinking women (those consuming more than 21 units per week). A total of 7% of all men and 4% of all women were concerned about their drinking even though their weekly consumption was below the limit set for excessive drinking in the study.

99

The World Health Organization *(267)* has developed a simple instrument termed AUDIT to screen for people with early signs of alcohol-related problems (Fig. 20 and 21). The WHO core screening instrument consists of ten simple questions, seven of them chosen because they were the most representative of the following signs:

— alcohol dependence and black-outs (4 questions);

— negative reactions to alcohol (1 question);

— alcohol problems (2 questions).

The other three questions are about consumption. The instrument has been shown to be reliable in six different countries. Its validity was calculated for drinking patients, using as the criterion for a positive case a hazardous alcohol consumption defined as a mean daily alcohol intake of 40 g or more for men or 20 g or more for women. Its sensitivity had a mean value of 80% and was higher in men than in women while its specificity, with a mean value of 89%, was higher in women than in men. The mean positive predictive value was 60% and the mean negative predictive value 95%. The WHO instrument also includes a clinical screening programme procedure consisting of a two-question trauma history, a brief clinical examination and a blood test.

Self-Assessment Questionnaires and Biological Markers

The Malmö Preventive Programme *(268–274)* was able to demonstrate that a combination of questionnaire responses and biological test results was highly predictive of future alcohol-related death: GGT concentration and the Mm-MAST score had strong positive correlations; serum creatinine had a strong inverse correlation; and total serum cholesterol had a less strong inverse correlation. Using a logistic analysis of the answers to the Mm-MAST questionnaire, the serum GGT values and the inverse values of serum creatinine, it could be shown that the higher the values in this logistic score, the higher the probability of alcohol-related death.

Instruments for assessing dependence
Since the alcohol-dependence syndrome was first described, a number of questionnaires have been developed to assess its severity. The first such instrument was the Severity of Alcohol Dependence Questionnaire (SADQ) *(276)* which has subsequently been revised and shortened to 20 items *(277,278)* (Fig. 22).

This questionnaire has been tested for reliability, construct and concurrent validity. It grades the severity of alcohol dependence on a continuous scale, taking into account the severity of the syndrome. No attempt is made to classify subjects as "dependent" or "not dependent"; rather they are assigned to one of a number of grades of dependence.

100

Fig. 20. The WHO core screening instrument

Please circle the answer that is correct for you.

1. How often do you have a drink* containing alcohol?

| NEVER | MONTHLY OR LESS | 2–4 TIMES A MONTH | 2–3 TIMES A WEEK | 4 OR MORE TIMES A WEEK |

2. How many drinks containing alcohol do you have on a typical day when you are drinking?

| 1 OR 2 | 3 OR 4 | 5 OR 6 | 7–9 | 10 OR MORE |

3. How often do you have 6 or more drinks on one occasion?

| NEVER | LESS THAN MONTHLY | MONTHLY | WEEKLY | DAILY OR ALMOST DAILY |

4. How often during the last year have you found it difficult to get the thought of alcohol out of your mind?

| NEVER | LESS THAN MONTHLY | MONTHLY | WEEKLY | DAILY OR ALMOST DAILY |

5. How often during the last year have you found that you were not able to stop drinking once you had started?

| NEVER | LESS THAN MONTHLY | MONTHLY | WEEKLY | DAILY OR ALMOST DAILY |

6. How often during the last year have you been unable to remember what happened the night before because you had been drinking?

| NEVER | LESS THAN MONTHLY | MONTHLY | WEEKLY | DAILY OR ALMOST DAILY |

7. How often during the last year have you needed a first drink in the morning to get yourself going after a heavy drinking session?

| NEVER | LESS THAN MONTHLY | MONTHLY | WEEKLY | DAILY OR ALMOST DAILY |

8. How often during the last year have you had a feeling of guilt or remorse after drinking?

| NEVER | LESS THAN MONTHLY | MONTHLY | WEEKLY | DAILY OR ALMOST DAILY |

9. Have you or someone else been injured as a result of your drinking?

| NO | YES, BUT NOT IN THE LAST YEAR | YES, DURING THE LAST YEAR |

10. Has a relative or friend or a doctor or other health worker, been concerned about your drinking or suggested you cut down?

| NO | YES, BUT NOT IN THE LAST YEAR | YES, DURING THE LAST YEAR |

---

* One drink is (give national examples).

Source: Saunders & Aasland (267).

101

Fig. 21. Scoring for the WHO core screening instrument

Item 1:	Never	= 0
	Monthly or less	= 1
	2–4 times a month	= 2
	2–3 times a week	= 3
	4 or more times a week	= 4
Item 2:	1–2 drinks	= 0
	3–4 drinks	= 1
	5–6 drinks	= 2
	7–9 drinks	= 3
	10+ drinks	= 4
Items 3–8:	Never	= 0
	Less than monthly	= 1
	Monthly	= 2
	Weekly	= 3
	Daily or almost daily	= 4
Items 9 & 10:	No	= 0
	Yes, but not in the last year	= 2
	Yes, during the last year	= 4

The maximum possible score is 40.

Source: Saunders & Aasland *(267)*.

Scores on the SADQ correlate with indices of withdrawal symptom severity as assessed by a physician in patients attending a detoxification unit. Further research is in progress to discover whether the SADQ is capable of predicting alcoholism treatment outcome.

Biological indicators
Biological indicators of alcohol consumption are likely to be more objective than questionnaires. One such indicator is raised GGT, which has proved to be one of the most sensitive tests for early liver disorder. The exact mechanism underlying the rise is not known, but it is assumed to be related to enzyme induction. GGT has been reported to be raised in 60–80% of clinic sample populations. However, Kristenson & Trell *(256)* showed that a raised GGT was not a sensitive indicator of alcoholism in a health screening investigation that identified only one third of the subjects as alcoholics. High levels of this enzyme may also be caused by barbiturates and other drugs, or other forms of liver disease unrelated to alcohol. An excess of false-positive readings may therefore be observed in clinic populations. Raised levels begin to return to normal after 48 hours of abstention, which makes the timing of sample collection critical.

Enlargement of the red corpuscles without anaemia is often found in excessive drinkers, and a raised mean corpuscular volume (MCV) is now a widely used indicator of harmful drinking. The MCV is raised in 50–60% of sample clinic populations. It is an abnormality that is not corrected by folate supplements.

Neither of these tests is very reliable for screening purposes: they are not particularly sensitive and lack power, having too high a false-positive rate. In a working population, excluding men with other causes of raised values, 50% who admit drinking over 56 units a week have a GGT of more than 50 IU per litre (false-positives 15%) and 23–32% have an MCV over 98 (false-positives 5%) *(275)*.

Case Identification

Primary health care provides a number of opportunities to screen for abnormal consumption by questionnaire. For instance, many primary health care facilities register their patients formally when they attend for the first time, and both clinical and social data can be obtained from these newly registered patients. This can be done by various methods: either by inviting the patients back for a special appointment, by having them interviewed by nurses or other staff, by asking them to fill in a questionnaire, or by giving them a computer-based interview *(279)*. In many primary care systems also, registered patients are systematically invited to attend for health checks, usually as part of screening or health promotion programmes *(280)*.

In the United Kingdom — to take an example — two thirds of the population registered with a primary health care service consult that service within a one-year period, and nine tenths within a five-year period. If all individuals attending were asked to complete a health questionnaire, over time most of the practice-based population could be fully screened.

A health questionnaire can also be mailed, with a freepost return envelope, to all registered patients or to all patients residing within a defined community. Although such mailings are costly, response rates of up to 75% can be achieved *(281)*.

A consultation may itself suggest that a patient is at high risk of alcohol-related problems, in which case further information can be ascertained either from previous records or data bases, or indirectly from the patient *(282,283)*. The factors that should alert health staff are as follows.

1.   A family history of alcohol-related problems. This association is very important when the spouse is known to drink heavily.

2.   Membership of certain social groups. The primary health care team may have personal knowledge of heavy drinking circles locally, or of friendships that put the patient under group pressure to drink.

Fig. 22. Severity of Alcohol Dependence Questionnaire (SADQ)

AGE........................

SEX ....

First of all, we would like you to recall a recent month when you were drinking heavily in a way which, for you, was fairly typical of a heavy drinking period. Please fill in the month and the year.

MONTH .... YEAR ....

We would like to know more about your drinking during this time and during other periods when your drinking was similar. We want to know how often you experienced certain feelings. Please reply to each statement by putting a circle around ALMOST NEVER or SOMETIMES or OFTEN or NEARLY ALWAYS after each question.

PLEASE ANSWER EVERY QUESTION

First we want to know about the physical symptoms that you have experienced first thing in the morning during these typical periods of heavy drinking.

1. During a heavy drinking period, I wake up feeling sweaty.
    ALMOST NEVER   SOMETIMES   OFTEN   NEARLY ALWAYS

2. During a heavy drinking period, my hands shake first thing in the morning.
    ALMOST NEVER   SOMETIMES   OFTEN   NEARLY ALWAYS

3. During a heavy drinking period, my whole body shakes violently first thing in the morning if I don't have a drink.
    ALMOST NEVER   SOMETIMES   OFTEN   NEARLY ALWAYS

4. During a heavy drinking period, I wake up absolutely drenched in sweat.
    ALMOST NEVER   SOMETIMES   OFTEN   NEARLY ALWAYS

The following statements refer to moods and states of mind you may have experienced first thing in the morning during these periods of heavy drinking.

5. When I'm drinking heavily, I dread waking up in the morning.
    ALMOST NEVER   SOMETIMES   OFTEN   NEARLY ALWAYS

6. During a heavy drinking period, I am frightened of meeting people first thing in the morning.
    ALMOST NEVER   SOMETIMES   OFTEN   NEARLY ALWAYS

7. During a heavy drinking period, I feel at the edge of despair when I awake.
    ALMOST NEVER   SOMETIMES   OFTEN   NEARLY ALWAYS

8. During a heavy drinking period, I feel very frightened when I awake.
    ALMOST NEVER   SOMETIMES   OFTEN   NEARLY ALWAYS

104

The following statements also refer to the recent period when your drinking was heavy, and to periods like it.

9. During a heavy drinking period, I like to have a morning drink.

ALMOST NEVER   SOMETIMES   OFTEN   NEARLY ALWAYS

10. During a heavy drinking period, I always gulp my first few morning drinks down as quickly as possible.

ALMOST NEVER   SOMETIMES   OFTEN   NEARLY ALWAYS

11. During a heavy drinking period, I drink in the morning to get rid of the shakes.

ALMOST NEVER   SOMETIMES   OFTEN   NEARLY ALWAYS

12. During a heavy drinking period, I have a very strong craving for a drink when I awake.

ALMOST NEVER   SOMETIMES   OFTEN   NEARLY ALWAYS

Again the following statements refer to the recent period of heavy drinking and the periods like it.

13. During a heavy drinking period, I drink more than a quarter of a bottle of spirits per day (4 doubles or 1 bottle of wine or 4 pints of beer).

ALMOST NEVER   SOMETIMES   OFTEN   NEARLY ALWAYS

14. During a heavy drinking period, I drink more than half a bottle of spirits per day (or 2 bottles of wine or 8 pints of beer).

ALMOST NEVER   SOMETIMES   OFTEN   NEARLY ALWAYS

15. During a heavy drinking period, I drink more than one bottle of spirits per day (or 4 bottles of wine or 15 pints of beer).

ALMOST NEVER   SOMETIMES   OFTEN   NEARLY ALWAYS

16. During a heavy drinking period, I drink more than two bottle of spirits per day (or 8 bottles of wine or 30 pints of beer).

ALMOST NEVER   SOMETIMES   OFTEN   NEARLY ALWAYS

IMAGINE THE FOLLOWING SITUATION:

     (1) You have been COMPLETELY off drink for a FEW WEEKS.

     (2) You then drink VERY HEAVILY for TWO DAYS.

HOW WOULD YOU FEEL THE MORNING AFTER THOSE TWO DAYS OF HEAVY DRINKING?

17. I would start to sweat.

NOT AT ALL   SLIGHTLY   MODERATELY   QUITE A LOT

18. My hands would shake.

NOT AT ALL   SLIGHTLY   MODERATELY   QUITE A LOT

19. My body would shake.

NOT AT ALL   SLIGHTLY   MODERATELY   QUITE A LOT

20. I would be craving for a drink.

NOT AT ALL   SLIGHTLY   MODERATELY   QUITE A LOT

Source: Stockwell et al. *(277)*.

3. An interest in beer or wine drinking as a hobby. This should alert staff to ask about consumption.

4. The opportunity for heavy, unsupervised drinking or for obtaining alcohol cheaply and easily as a result of the patient's occupation. Primary health care physicians themselves are a very high-risk group.

5. A lack of firm social roots and supports, and deviation from social norms.

6. Prominent family or other problems. Families with known psychological or social difficulties place their members at high risk of problems related to alcohol.

7. Obesity, particularly in men. This has a strong correlation with high consumption of alcohol.

8. A smell of alcohol on the breath. This is undoubtedly the most common alerting factor, although signs of intoxication such as mood lability, uninhibited behaviour and ataxia may also be present without there being any obvious smell of alcohol. These other signs may also indicate intoxication due to drugs, or to a combination of alcohol and other drugs.

Some patients may present directly either with concerns about their drinking or with disorders that have already been caused by it. In such cases, the points to look for are as follows.

1. Indirect allusions. Only a small proportion of patients will make a direct inquiry about their drinking and express their fears about it. Usually the approach will be indirect, or the spouse or another member of the family may broach the subject. There is a social stigma connected with alcohol problems, and people will often test the tolerance of professional staff before risking a direct request for help.

2. Blackouts, collapses, fits and "turns". Alcohol can provoke these signs, which may be due to ataxia, vasovagal disturbance, withdrawal, hypoglycaemia or acute overdose and toxicity.

3. Physical damage. Any individual presenting with any of the forms of physical damage outlined on pp. 54–59 should be asked about his or her alcohol consumption. The presence of several problems and a pattern linked with a history of risky drinking is highly significant.

4. Accidents and trauma. Heavy drinkers are prone to injury and may present to primary health care services or to accident and emergency departments. Road traffic accidents and injuries sustained during fights are particularly important.

5. Psychological conditions. Insomnia is often associated with the heavy use of alcohol, and anyone presenting with feelings of depression

or anxiety, or with phobias, particularly needs to be assessed for alcohol consumption. In addition, acute psychosis during withdrawal, pathological jealousy and possessiveness, and the persistent use of tranquillizers and hypnotics are all associated with heavy drinking.

6. Physical and psychological abuse of members of the family. There is a strong association between these two factors and heavy drinking; furthermore, heavy drinkers may induce symptoms of anxiety, depression and behavioural disorder in close relations. Separation and divorce are commonly both the cause and effect of heavy drinking.

7. Haematological and biochemical information. The patient's medical record will contain information that can alert staff to the need for fuller assessment. Indices such as MCV and GGT can indicate probable damage due to alcohol.

The importance of these checklists in alerting staff to the possibility that alcohol is the underlying cause of the consultation is illustrated by a study by Wilkins in the United Kingdom (263). Using an at-risk register, Wilkins noted in his primary health care practice that during a period of one year 5% of the registered adult population consulted the practice because of one of the at-risk characteristics. Of the 546 patients at risk, 28% were found to have problems associated with alcohol compared to only 3% of those who consulted but had no at-risk characteristics.

Classification
The Royal College of General Practitioners (RCGP) in the United Kingdom (36) has devised a method of classifying patients who are at risk because of their drinking (Fig. 23). Individuals are assigned to one of three groups according to their consumption: those who drink little or none (women, 15 units or under weekly; men, 20 units or under weekly); those who have a high consumption (women, over 30 units weekly; men, over 50 units weekly); and those who fall in between, the intermediate group. This classification is intended as a guide for members of the primary health care team, to help them monitor risk from alcohol, assess the risk and any damage already done, and plan suitable follow-up schemes.

Vulnerability
However, not everyone is equally vulnerable to the same amount of alcohol. Women are at risk of liver disease at lower levels of consumption than men, and people in the following groups should be considered to be at higher risk than their consumption alone would indicate:

— children and the very old; and

— people subject to additive or synergistic factors, including those with chronic conditions such as epilepsy, raised blood sugar and

107

Fig. 23. Action for patients in different drinking categories

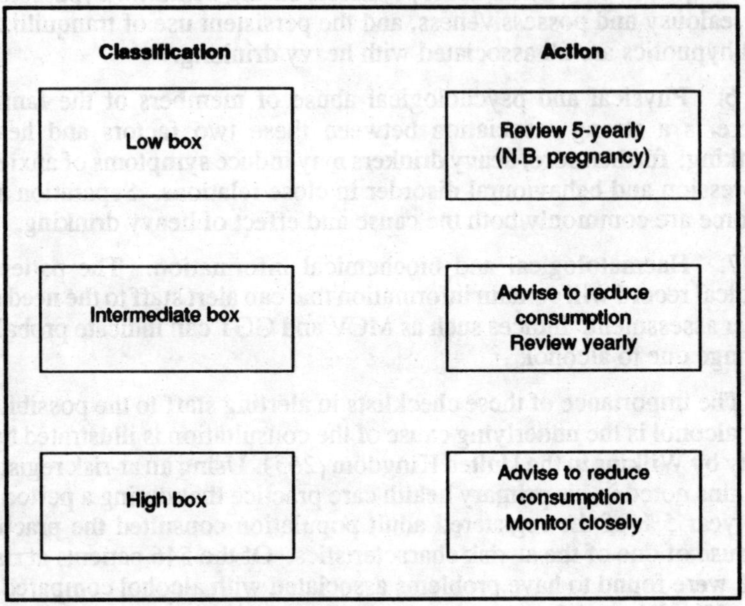

Classification	Action
Low box	Review 5-yearly (N.B. pregnancy)
Intermediate box	Advise to reduce consumption Review yearly
High box	Advise to reduce consumption Monitor closely

Source: Royal College of General Practitioners *(36)*.

raised blood pressure; those with psychological difficulties such as anxiety and depression; those who are taking medication that interacts with alcohol; and those with potentially harmful lifestyles, including cigarette smokers and people who are overweight.

Assessment

People in the RCGP intermediate group who have one of the vulnerability factors listed above, and all individuals in the RCGP high group, require a fuller assessment (Fig. 24), the primary objective of which should be to obtain and also to give information so that decisions can be made about management. Information seeking alone may not work and many high-risk drinkers are likely to feel threatened by it. A full assessment, however, can be therapeutic in itself: the drinker may be helped, possibly for the first time, to consider both the drinking and its effects, and may even think about making some decisions without specific advice having been offered. On the other hand, some people are unwilling or unable to be honest; guilt, fear or confusion interfere, so that the problems seem too distressing to contemplate. In such cases the primary health care worker needs to draw back and deal with the blocks rather than prod insistently at raw areas, which may cause the drinker to build up even more solid defences.

The assessment must also indicate the starting point, which means that it must reveal what social, psychological and physical damage has been done and how much of it can be corrected (Table 28). The assessment should also help the assessor to understand why the person drinks in the way he or she does, and should throw light on both the drinker's and other family members' attitudes to drinking, which may include such features as the following.

1. Misunderstandings (lack of knowledge, incorrect knowledge or myths) or denial, which make the benefits seem much more real than the remote possibility of harm.

2. Periods of indecision, often over many years, during which individuals vacillate between accepting that their drinking is harmful and that they ought to do something about it, and non-acceptance or denial, with attempts to fix blame on anyone and anything but themselves.

3. Practical problems during periods of change, when drinkers may receive all sorts of advice from professionals and lay people, much of it conflicting (cut down/give up completely; stay at home/go into a specialist unit; take this drug/don't touch it).

Before the risk of damage can be estimated, it is necessary to find out and record the number of units of alcohol the person typically consumes per week, by asking about the kind of drink taken, the frequency with which it is drunk, and the amount consumed on each occasion. It may be helpful to ask about the cost of the person's drinking, as a cross-check and also as a measure of social damage. If the drinker finds it difficult to respond to these questions, the interviewer should ask about the last drink taken and then lead on to more general inquiries.

If a person is reluctant to talk about his or her drinking at all, it may be necessary to explain why the interviewer is interested in it in medical or preventive terms, and to see if the drinker can offer any reasons for the reluctance. If the reluctance persists, it is usually a mistake to continue because the person may retreat into evasion and untruth; the reluctance should simply be noted and the interviewer should return to the subject on another occasion.

The past history of drinking is vital, and for those in whom drinking is highly likely to cause damage it is essential to discover when the drinking started and what events it was linked to. Drinking often escalates at a time of separation or loss; furthermore, heavy drinking may persist even after the original reason for it has diminished in importance, often because the drinking itself has caused more problems, perhaps

Fig. 24. Alcohol card

Alcohol Card			
SURNAME	FORENAMES	D of B	SEX
DATE	ETHNIC ORIGIN		
PRESENTING PROBLEMS			
AMOUNT DRUNK/WEEK UNITS			
PATTERN OF DRINKING			
WHY MISUSING			
HARMS			
PHYSICAL			
PSYCHOLOGICAL			
BEHAVIOUR			
FAMILY			
SOCIAL			
RISK FACTORS			
OCCUPATION	PERSONALITY		
FAMILY	TOBACCO		
CULTURE	OTHER		
FAMILY	FAMILY OF ORIGIN		
MARITAL			
CHILDREN	CHILDHOOD		

Source: Tomson, O. (personal communication, 1986).

financially or at work. The history will need to explore this kind of vicious circle.

The history should also include information on any bouts of heavy drinking and what happened on the days before and after. What the person felt and thought, as well as his or her behaviour, is also important.

Finally, the interviewer should ask about previous attempts to cut down or abstain from alcohol, the events surrounding relapses, the

Fig. 24 (contd)

ATTEMPTS AT CONTROL	MAJOR ILLNESSES
	OTHER DRUGS

EXAMINATION	INVESTIGATIONS	
WT.	GGT	CHOL
	MCV	OTHER
B.P.	BAC	
	CREAT	
	URATE	

	DATE	DATE	DATE	DATE	DATE
PROBLEM NOT AGREED					
PROBLEM AGREED					
DECIDED ON ACTION					
ACTION IMPLEMENTED					

CONTRACT AND PLAN

ALCOHOL

HARM

FAMILY SEEN

DATE

CONTRACT

INVOLVED	
HV	MGC
SW	AA
CAT	OTHER
ACS	
PSYCHOLOGIST	

attitudes and behaviour of those close to the drinker, and a little about the drinker's early life and upbringing.

Physical assessment should include the measurement of pulse, blood pressure, height and weight, and a search for signs of liver disease. Other bodily systems can be examined if the history indicates possible damage.

Biological tests for evidence of impairment of function (which will act as a baseline for later monitoring) should include haemoglobin, mean

111

Table 28. Alcohol problems checklist

Health problems

Stomach upsets? ....   Indigestion? ....

Sickness, vomiting? ....   Diarrhoea, loose bowels? ....

Difficulty sleeping? ....   Tiredness/difficulty
                              concentrating? ....

Easily upset? ....

Depressed? ....

Social problems

Arguments at home about drinking? ....

Arguments at home made worse by drinking? ....

Family member threatened to leave because of drinking? ....

Been asked to leave pub/party, etc. because drunk? ....

Money worries because of drinking? ....

Problems with police because of drinking? ....

Accidents/work problems

Trouble at work because of drinking? ....

Absence from work because of drinking? ....

Been in accident because of drinking? ....

Symptoms of developing tolerance

Unable to keep a drink limit? ....

Difficulty preventing getting drunk? ....

Restless without a drink? ....

Trembling after drinking the day before? ....

Drinking in the morning? ....

Table 29. Normal range of values for laboratory tests

Test	Range
Haemoglobin	
Men	13.5 – 18.0 g/dl
Women	11.5 – 16.0 g/dl
Mean corpuscular volume	76 – 96 fl
Erythrocyte sedimentation rate	
Men	1–10 mm/hour
Women	0 –15 mm/hour
White blood count	$4.0 - 11.0 \times 10^9$/litre
α-Glutaryltranspeptidase	15 – 40 IU/litre
Creatinine	70 –150 µmol/litre
Alkaline phosphatase	100 – 300 IU/litre
Bilirubin	3 –17 µmol/litre
Proteins	60 – 80 g/litre

corpuscular volume, erythrocyte sedimentation rate, white blood count, α-glutaryltranspeptidase, creatinine, alkaline phosphatase, bilirubin and proteins. Blood and breath alcohol test results can be added to the dossier if available. Normal values for the tests mentioned vary from one laboratory to another, but a normal range is given in Table 29 above.

7

Management

The primary health care team's response to patients must be tailored to the level of drinking and/or the problems of each individual. People who are drinking at low-risk levels will need only a fairly brief intervention, but those who are at greater risk or already have definite problems require more intensive treatment. There is evidence that intervention in primary health care is effective, and various models of therapy are available.

Prognosis and Treatment of Advanced Alcohol Problems

The prognosis for patients with advanced alcohol problems is generally unfavourable (194,195,284). Their mortality rate over a five-year period can be up to between four and ten times that of age- and sex-matched controls from the general population. By the time they present to health care facilities, many have already suffered severe social disruption and damage to their health.

In most developed countries, specialized inpatient units have been established in response to these people's needs, but despite the considerable investment made there is little evidence that such services are cost-effective (285,286). Indeed, most studies have failed to show any benefit from various types of intervention for patients with advanced problems. Intensive treatment programmes have the disadvantage that they tend to perpetuate the belief that "alcoholics" are a separate group of people requiring special and complicated treatment. The effect of this has been to draw attention away from individuals with less severe alcohol problems, who numerically are a far more significant group and, as already stated, make the major contribution to the public health problem of alcohol. In recent years, as a result, the emphasis has shifted towards intervening at an earlier stage in the drinker's career.

The effectiveness of minimal intervention

There is considerable evidence of the benefit to be gained from minimal intervention in relation to both smoking and drinking.

A number of researchers have evaluated the effect of general practitioners' advice on the smoking behaviour of their patients (287,288). In the study by Russell et al. (287) one group was given simple but firm advice to stop smoking, during a routine consultation. Another group was given the same advice, warned that there would be follow up, and provided with a four-page information leaflet entitled *How you can give up smoking*. A third group of controls was given neither advice nor information. Follow-up data were obtained at one month and one year after the consultation. The results showed that motivation and the intention to stop smoking were increased in the group given advice only, as was the proportion of patients who attempted to stop. At one-year follow-up, 5.0% of those in the group given the smokers' information leaflet had stopped smoking, compared to 0.3% in the control group and 3.3% in the advice only group. Light smokers were more likely to stop successfully than heavy smokers. There were also pronounced differences in the success rates achieved by different doctors.

Although the effects of the programme were not dramatic, it was concluded that if all general practitioners in Britain were to adopt the simple measure of providing the leaflet, the intervention could produce half a million ex-smokers in one year.

Malmö Project, Sweden

Kristenson et al. in Malmö (289) studied a group of 585 healthy middle-aged men (aged 46–49) who had been identified as heavy drinkers during a general health screening project. They used GGT levels as a preliminary screening test, and then enrolled the top 10% of the distribution in the study. Of those who had a raised GGT on two occasions three weeks apart, 76% were found to be either heavy or moderate drinkers. Heavy drinking was defined as more than 40 g of alcohol per day and moderate as 20–40 g per day.

The sample with raised GGT were randomly divided into an intervention group and a control group. The control group were simply informed by letter that they had impaired liver function, advised to cut down on their drinking, and invited for new liver tests after two years. The intervention group were given a detailed physical examination and interviewed about their drinking history, symptoms of alcohol dependence and any evidence of alcohol-related problems. They were then offered appointments with the same physician every third month, and monthly appointments with the same nurse, who repeated the GGT test on each occasion. They were also advised to moderate their drinking. This group was able to monitor their progress because they were regularly told what their GGT levels were and were encouraged to try to return to

116

normal. Once their test results had reached an acceptable level, the frequency of clinical contact was reduced.

The progress of all the subjects was evaluated two and four years after the initial screening. After four years, the GGT values of both groups had decreased significantly. There were, however, important differences between the two groups in terms of sickness absenteeism, hospitalization and mortality. In the intervention group, the mean number of sick days per person had increased from 24 to 29, while in the control group it had risen from 25 to 52 days. The control group as a whole had spent 1644 days in hospital over the four-year period, but the intervention group only 808 days. If alcohol-related conditions were isolated from other causes of hospitalization, the difference was even more striking: 482 days for alcohol-related conditions in the control group as opposed to 133 in the intervention group, a ratio of 3 to 1. Finally, it was noted that after five years there had been twice as many deaths in the control group as in the intervention group. This study showed that simple intervention based on regular feedback about a biochemical marker can have significant effects on the drinking habits and physical health of a population.

Edinburgh Royal Infirmary Project, Scotland
In Edinburgh, Chick et al. *(290)* studied the effectiveness of a brief intervention used for heavy drinkers identified in a general hospital as having a current alcohol problem. The actual presence of the problem was established by a nurse, using a structured interview lasting 10 minutes and covering drinking habits, recent and previous medical history, and social background. MCV and GGT were recorded for each patient. Any patient found to have an unexplained raised MCV and denying having alcohol problems was reinterviewed. The criteria for inclusion in the study were that the patient should not have received prior treatment for an alcohol problem, and should have some degree of social stability to facilitate follow-up. The patient also had to show evidence of heavy drinking or alcohol-related problems when questioned about:

— alcohol consumption patterns;

— current medical problems (alcohol-related);

— past medical problems (alcohol-related);

— symptoms of alcohol dependence; and

— alcohol-related social problems.

The heavy drinkers identified by the interview were randomly divided into two groups. No comment was made to the control group, although all agreed to be followed up one year later. Each member of the intervention group received a further 30–60 minutes' counselling from the nurse, in the presence of the patient's spouse. Finally, the patient was

117

given a booklet suggesting techniques for cutting down. The outcome after one year is shown in Table 30.

The DRAMS Scheme
Sixteen general practitioners participated in a controlled trial of the Scottish Health Education Group's DRAMS (Drinking Reasonably and Moderately with Self-control) Scheme *(291)*. The scheme was evaluated by randomly assigning 104 heavy or problem drinkers to three groups: a group participating in the DRAMS scheme (N=34), a group given simple advice only (N=32) and a non-intervention group (N=38). Six-month follow-up information was obtained for 91 subjects. For the sample as a whole, there was a significant reduction in alcohol consumption, a significant improvement on a measure of physical health and wellbeing, and significant reductions in GGT and MCV. However, there were no significant differences between the groups in reduction of alcohol consumption, although patients in the DRAMS group did show a significantly greater reduction in GGT than patients in the group receiving advice only. Only 14 patients in the DRAMS group completed the full DRAMS procedure. The main drawback to the study was that the sample size was too small to permit confirmation of the hypothesis that there was no difference between the three groups.

The MRC Study
The aim of the Medical Research Council of the United Kingdom's General Practice Research Framework Study on Lifestyle and Health was to determine the effectiveness of advice from general practitioners to heavy drinkers on how to cut down *(292)*. The study was carried out in 47 group practices in the United Kingdom. Initial screening of 62 153 patients aged 17 to 69 using a health survey questionnaire was followed by an interview, after which 917 heavy drinkers (men drinking at least 35 units a week and women drinking at least 21 units) were assigned at random to either treatment or control groups. Patients in the treatment group were interviewed by their general practitioner, given advice and information on how to reduce their consumption, and followed up every third month. At one year, a mean reduction in consumption of 18 units per week had occurred among the treated men, compared with 8 units among the male controls. Some 44% fewer men were drinking heavily in the treatment group, compared with 26% fewer in the control group. A mean reduction in weekly consumption of 12 units occurred among treated women, compared to 6 units among controls, while 48% fewer women were drinking heavily in the treatment group, compared with 29% fewer in the control group.

The mean GGT value dropped significantly more in the treated men — by 2.4 IU — compared to the controls, in whom it had dropped by 1.1 IU. The reduction in both consumption and GGT levels increased with the number of interventions by the general practitioner. On the basis

**Table 30. Effectiveness of treatment
(minimal intervention)**

Result after one year	Controls (N)	Treatment (N)
Dead	2	1
Refused/no contact	12	8
Blood tests incomplete	5	5
Blood tests complete:		
Improved	20	34
Not improved	39	31

Source: Chick et al. *(290)*.

of the results, the investigators calculated that advice from general practitioners in the United Kingdom could each year result in a reduction to moderate levels of the alcohol consumption of 210 000 men and 130 000 women who are currently drinking more than they should.

The Therapeutic Response

Low-risk drinkers
Patients assessed as being at minimum risk will for the time being require little or no further action so far as their drinking is concerned. One must remember, however, that this may change; people sometimes become more vulnerable as time goes by, even without a change in their drinking habits, because of other events in their lives. Low-risk drinkers should be invited to come back for a further health check in five years' time, when their consumption can be assessed again.

Moderate-risk drinkers
Drinkers who are at moderate risk are a very important group, being responsible for the majority of the alcohol-related problems that occur in a society. These people can be identified in general practice and offered advice on how to cut down; at this stage the advice will very likely be effective, and prevent them from moving into the higher-risk category. Moderate-risk drinkers who have one or more of the vulnerability factors (p. 107) should be treated as being at high risk.

Most moderate-risk drinkers need advice on how to reduce their consumption to a safe level, that is below 20 units for men and 15 units for women weekly; some suggestions are given in Table 31. The

119

Table 31. Components of minimal intervention

1. *Ask patients what they think about their drinking*

2. *Summarize assessment findings*

   (a) weekly consumption
   (b) current effects on physical health
   (c) current effects on life at home or at work
   (d) evidence of tolerance

3. *Discuss results of laboratory tests*

   (a) GGT
   (b) MCV

   (Emphasize that any harmful effects which may have occurred are almost certainly fully reversible if patient reduces consumption)

4. *Indicate patient's position on histogram*

   Show that the patient's consumption is considerably above the "normal range", even though it may appear quite moderate within the patient's own social/drinking circle

5. *Give information on risks of heavy drinking*

   Mention: being overweight
   stomach upsets
   liver disease
   headaches, hangover
   difficulty in sleeping
   sexual difficulties

6. *Give information on advantages of drinking less*

   Mention: financial savings
   safer driving

7. *Give patient a copy of "That's the limit" or "Drams pack"*

   Inform the patient that the booklets give further information on:

   (a) risks of heavy drinking
   (b) how to calculate alcohol consumption
   (c) safe limits of consumption for men and women
   (d) suggestions about how to reduce consumption

8. *Advise patient to cut down on drinking and give diary pack*

   (a) Tell patient that this is a form of prescription
   (b) Indicate that the limits you recommend are:
   not more than 20 units/week for men
   not more than 15 units/week for women

9. *Give patient follow-up appointment (2 weeks)*

   (a) Ask patient to fill in drinking record cards for the two weeks
   (b) Emphasize that you believe it is important for patient to attend
   (c) Explain that you will in any case ask about alcohol consumption at
   next attendance

interviewer should first explore the patient's general beliefs about drinking and health, and then discuss the patient's own consumption level and any harm it may be doing — not only its health effects but also its effects on home and work life. It is particularly important to relate excessive drinking to the patient's presenting complaint, where applicable. It is a good idea, too, to demonstrate that the patient's consumption is above the normal range, even though it may appear quite moderate within his or her drinking circle. This can be done by using an alcohol histogram that indicates the distribution of alcohol consumption among the population for men and for women (Fig. 25 and 26). The interviewer can also tell the patient about such risks of heavy drinking as becoming overweight, stomach upsets, liver disease, headaches and hangovers, anxiety and depression, sexual difficulties and difficulty in sleeping.

The patient's attention should be drawn to the advantages of drinking less — saving money and safer driving, for example. Self-help booklets, if available, are a good adjunct to spoken advice; these usually include information on the risks of heavy drinking, how to calculate consumption in terms of units, sensible limits of consumption for women and men, and suggestions on how to cut down. Some examples are the Scottish Health Education Group's DRAMS pack, the English Health Education Authority's *That's the limit*, and the Dutch and English *Cut down on drinking* booklets. It is important to recommend and keep repeating the sensible upper limits to consumption (15 units weekly for women and 20 units for men), and to emphasize that these amounts should be spread over the whole week rather than concentrated into bouts or binges.

High-risk drinkers
The aim in treating someone who is drinking heavily or who has alcohol-related problems is to reduce the patient's consumption and relieve the harm it is causing.

People undergoing treatment for high-risk drinking pass through three stages: pre-understanding, understanding and action *(293)*. At the pre-understanding stage they have not thought about their drinking being harmful, and need help to understand the relationship between consumption and damage. At the understanding stage they have thought about their drinking, but not done anything about it; they need help with decision-making and with weighing up and altering the balance sheet of the good and bad effects of drinking. At the action stage they are actually trying to do something about their drinking and may need help with the process of change. The aim of therapy is to help high-risk drinkers move from pre-understanding through understanding to action; the therapist's exact response will depend on which stage the person has reached at that point.

The first step to understanding is for the drinker to receive feedback from a diary on how much he or she is drinking. The drinking diary itself is an important part of the therapy. Many people are surprised at how

121

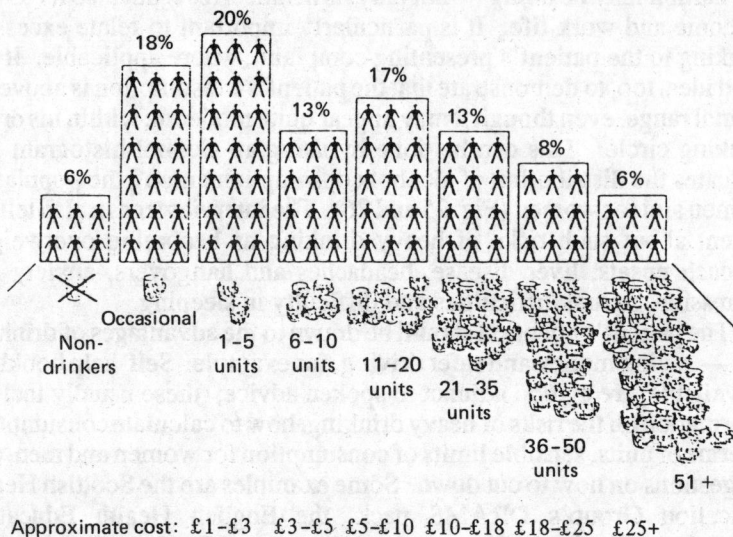

Fig. 25. Distribution and approximate cost of units of alcohol consumed weekly by men (England & Wales)

Non-drinkers 6%
Occasional 18%
1-5 units 20%
6-10 units 13%
11-20 units 17%
21-35 units 13%
36-50 units 8%
51+ 6%

Approximate cost: £1-£3   £3-£5 £5-£10 £10-£18 £18-£25 £25+

Source: Wallace, P. & Haines, A. (personal communication from Epidemiology and Medical Care Unit, Northwick Park Hospital, 1986).

quickly the diary adds up and how much alcohol they actually do consume in a week.

The next step is for therapist and patient to list any problems the patient has that may possibly be related to drink. Some of these problems will already be apparent, or documented in the medical notes. Making a list of them may help the patient to realize for the first time how some symptoms are related to alcohol, and to accept that an adjustment in drinking habits is necessary. The list can be particularly effective if the symptoms are immediately aggravated by drinking and so act as a reminder of the need for a change. If the presenting symptom can also be related to alcohol, this too will have immediate and powerful impact.

The patient who has begun to understand the harm or potential harm his or her heavy drinking is causing may still need help in deciding whether or not to do anything about it. It may be obvious to an outsider that the patient should drink less but it can still be difficult for the patient to grasp this idea. The therapist can help by drawing up a balance sheet of the advantages and disadvantages of drinking, discussing each of them in turn and attempting to tip the balance in favour of cutting down (see also p. 32).

122

Fig, 26. Distribution and approximate cost of units of alcohol consumed weekly by women (England & Wales)

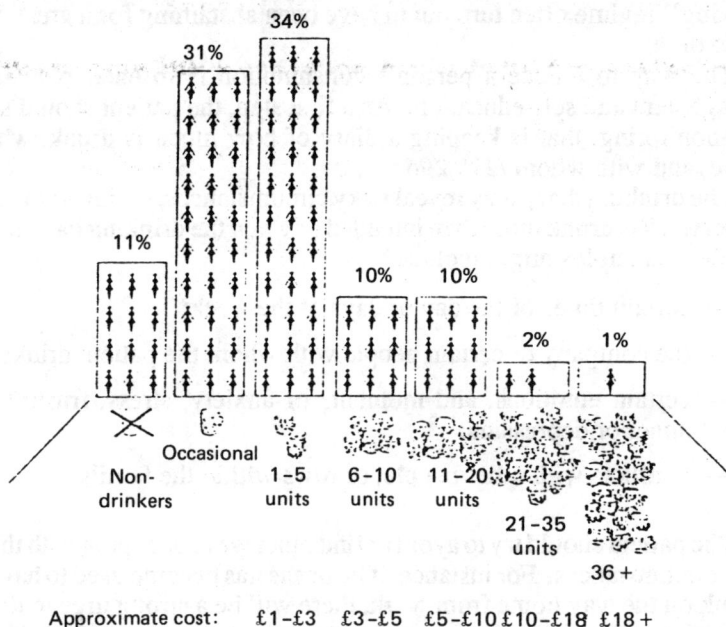

34%

31%

11%

10%   10%

2%   1%

Non-drinkers   Occasional   1-5 units   6-10 units   11-20 units   21-35 units   36+

Approximate cost: £1-£3   £3-£5   £5-£10 £10-£18   £18+

Source: Wallace, P. & Haines, A. (personal communication from Epidemiology and Medical Care Unit, Northwick Park Hospital, 1986).

At this stage, the first thing is to find out what the patient wants and to reach agreement or make a "contract" on the goals for change. Some people may need detoxification, which is discussed later.

The long-term goals will depend on the patient's previous history, the amount being drunk now, and the extent of the problems. If the drinking is very heavy, though so far harmless, the therapist can give advice on a sensible drinking level, as already discussed. Some drinkers with established problems will be able to drink less; however, there is evidence that it is better for people who have severe withdrawal symptoms or signs of severe physical damage, or who have systematically tried to control their drinking but without success, to aim at total abstinence *(294)*.

In practice, however, the early choice of an exact drinking goal may be less important than would at first appear. There are a variety of goals to choose from — for example, abstinence most of the time save for occasional "light" drinking; regular but "very light" drinking; or very

123

occasional "heavy" drinking. Furthermore, as treatment progresses and the individual's ideas and understanding develop, the preferred goal may also change. Indeed, people who have been following a "controlled drinking" regime often turn out to have been abstaining for a great deal of the time.

The way to reduce a person's consumption is to encourage self-management and self-education. As a first step, the patient should start self-monitoring, that is keeping a diary of how much is drunk, when, where, and with whom (295,296).

The drinking diary may reveal risky circumstances, or times at which the person has drunk more than intended or when the drinking has caused trouble. Examples might include:

— certain times of the day or days of the week;

— the company of certain people with whom the patient drinks;

— certain emotions, and moments of anxiety, stress, frustration, anger or depression:

— conflicts with other people, or rows within the family.

The patient should try to avoid or find other ways of coping with these risky circumstances. For instance, if he or she has become used to having a drink on the way home from work, there will be a strong urge to drink at that time. Heavy drinkers must learn to avoid situations where in the past they have drunk heavily, and confine their drinking to situations in which they have in the past drunk sensibly.

It is also helpful to suggest techniques for drinking less. Some useful tips are as follows.

• *Take non-alcoholic drinks.*

• *Take smaller sips.* Sip less often and take small sips. Count the number of sips it takes to finish a glass, and then try to increase the number for the next glass, and so on.

• *Occupy yourself.* Do something else that is enjoyable while you drink, to help distract your attention from the glass, and drink more slowly. Eat, for example, listen to music, play darts, talk, and so on.

• *Change the drink.* Changing the type of drink you take can help break old habits and reduce the amount you drink.

• *Drink for the taste.* Drink more slowly and enjoy the flavour.

• *Imitate the slow drinker.* Look round for someone who is drinking slowly and become a shadow, not picking up the glass until the other person does.

124

- *Put the glass down between sips.* If you hold the glass you will drink from it more often. Do something else with your hands instead of lifting the glass to your lips.

- *Dilute spirits.* Top up spirits with non-alcoholic mixers.

- *Reduce the amount you drink in "rounds".* Buy your own drinks, or buy one round and then go solo. When it is your round, do not buy yourself a drink. Order non-alcoholic drinks every so often.

- *Eat.* Eat before drinking or while drinking. Eating slows down the absorption of alcohol, and the fact of doing something else may reduce the amount you drink.

- *Take rest days.* Abstain from alcohol at least one day a week, or preferably two, three or even four days. Take up other forms of entertainment and relaxation.

- *Start later.* Start drinking later than usual; for example, go later to the pub.

- *Learn to refuse drinks.* Rehearse ways of refusing drinks: "No thanks, I'm cutting down", for example, or "Not tonight, I've got a bad stomach".

Once ways of cutting down have been discussed, doctor and patient must plan a realistic strategy for change. It is best to aim for specific short-term goals at first, rather than long-term goals and general intentions. This allows the patient to concentrate on the immediate future and gain a sense of achievement as each goal is reached.

Books are useful in that they reinforce the therapist's advice and inform the patient *(297)*. Self-help manuals can be used as an alternative to professional advice *(177,298)*.

Patients who give a history of severe withdrawal symptoms, or who show signs of withdrawal at the consultation, will need a period of detoxification and possibly help in dealing with the withdrawal symptoms. Detoxification can take place at home, in a general hospital, or in an alcohol treatment unit. It is now clear that many people can be detoxified at home, provided that there is a reasonably supportive family *(299)*.

The process of detoxification is very important in establishing a therapeutic relationship. The patient may feel vulnerable at this stage and is, of course, highly dependent on good health care. One or other member of the primary health care team, or someone from a specialized service — the community psychiatric nurse, for example — should visit the patient daily, not just to monitor the detoxification but also to build up the relationship. This is also a very favourable time for performing an assessment, not only of the patient but also of the rest of the family.

125

Diazepam is the preferred drug for detoxification. The starting dose and duration are determined by the anticipated severity of withdrawal, based on the previous withdrawal history. The pattern is likely to repeat that of previous withdrawals, unless the previous drinking was different in some way. It is important to make sure that the patient has not been using other drugs: tolerance to diazepam may have developed, which would indicate a longer regime at larger doses. For withdrawals at home which are expected to be severe, a maximum of 20 mg of diazepam four times a day, reduced daily and ending after seven days, may be necessary. In most cases much less is indicated. The medication should be closely supervised and the drug should preferably not be supplied in large quantities at a time.

If the patient gives a history of severe delirium tremens and/or withdrawal fits, or if his or her social circumstances are such that proper care is not available at home, then admission to hospital has to be considered.

Vitamins should be given during detoxification, intramuscularly or intravenously, daily for five days. Counselling of the family and the patient on the symptoms, signs, duration and management of detoxification helps to ensure a safe and constructive withdrawal.

To help maintain a lower level of drinking, it is essential to offer the patient follow-up. At follow-up the therapist should review progress, offer continuing help and support, and advise the patient on how to manage any difficulties. Progress should be reviewed regularly over a full year. The first six months often give a good idea of the longer-term prognosis.

Blood tests are useful for monitoring progress, and the results and their implications can be discussed with the patient. Their use in intervention has been demonstrated in the Malmö study referred to above *(289)*. GGT returns rapidly to normal with abstention, even as early as 48 hours after the last drink. A subsequent rise of 50% or more is strong evidence of further heavy drinking. Mean corpuscular volume, on the other hand, takes several weeks to return to normal after drinking is cut down. In the healthy person, alcohol is removed from the blood at a rate of about 15 mg per 100 ml per hour, and detectable blood concentrations are present for over 8 hours after the ingestion of three large beers. In patients with liver damage, concentrations may remain high for more than 24 hours.

Many heavy drinkers will have some form of relapse and need to be warned about this. They should be aware of the sort of problems likely to cause a relapse, and need to plan in advance so that they can deal with it and avoid situations where it is likely to occur *(300)*. It may be helpful for the patient, therapist and family to draw up a list of relapse precipitants. A relapse should not be regarded as a loss of all that has been achieved, but rather as an opportunity for the patient to learn how to cope with this kind of situation.

126

To help maintain their drinking at a lower level, some patients may need specific behavioural therapy managed by a clinical psychologist *(198)*. The type of therapy chosen will depend on the patient's reasons for drinking. Relaxation training, yoga or meditation may be helpful for people who drink in response to stress. Those who feel isolated or find it difficult to make friends sometimes benefit from social skills training. Some people need marital or family therapy if marital, family or sexual difficulties have preceded or resulted from their drinking. Others may need help in connection with their work, if the drinking has something to do with their occupation.

Sensitizing drugs can play a role in the management of heavy drinking where the goal is abstention, but their continued use demands a high degree of motivation on the part of the patient. Disulfiram (200 mg daily) is used to sensitize the body to alcohol; it causes flushing, headache, palpitations, nausea, faintness or collapse when alcohol is taken. The reaction can be severe, or even fatal, and disulfiram should not be prescribed for people with established cardiac, renal or hepatic disease, or those at risk of suicide. Liver function must be carefully monitored. Any patient using the drug on a long-term basis will need regular support; a family member or a friend can be very helpful.

Many studies have stressed the importance of family support *(301)*, including Saunders & Kershaw (see p. 69). Sometimes the therapist can help the family without even seeing the drinker, and it is not uncommon for changes in the family itself to cause the drinker to stop or cut down. There may be good reasons for seeing the family, or any member of it but the drinker; the therapist can help the family members deal with their own problems and change their own behaviour so that, rather than going on sustaining the drinker's drinking, they learn how to help the person either cut down or stop altogether.

The partners of heavy drinkers usually suffer greatly — socially, psychologically and physically. Many experience anxiety, sleeplessness, tension and depression. They often feel very guilty, and are full of self-blame. Some are obsessed with feelings of anger and punitiveness, which they vent on their children or their colleagues at work. Counselling helps them to cope with these feelings, and to avoid drink-sustaining behaviour within the family. It is important to listen and understand before attempting to help, and not to blame either partner for the problems.

Both partners should be encouraged to accept responsibility for their own behaviour, symptoms and feelings, and should be helped to make whatever changes seem desirable for the good of both. Their urge to change and their ability to change will depend on what stage of understanding they have reached.

Very often, the partner has been behaving in such a way that the drinker has been actively prevented from seeing what problems the drinking is causing. For example, the partner may have covered up by

127

making excuses for the drinker's avoidance of work, or by paying his or her debts. It may be only when the partner stops this cover-up that the drinker can face the reality of the situation.

The partner can also be encouraged to alter the balance sheet in favour of cutting down by rewarding non-drinking, and being careful not to reward drinking by taking the easy option and giving in to it. The right rewards help the drinker to change, so it is important for the partner to understand how he or she has in the past rewarded the drinking but punished non-drinking. For instance, a husband may nag his wife when she is sober again after a drinking bout — because he experiences this as an unpleasant sobriety; or a wife may pay more attention to her husband when he is drinking than when he is not. All this is part of an unhelpful reward structure which makes it more comfortable for the drinker to drink, even though at the same time the drinking discomforts the other partner.

While drinkers are in the process of changing, it is vital for their partners to encourage them; too often success is ignored, and failures severely punished. This can be a difficult time for a family who may have learned to cope without a fully functioning husband, father, wife or mother. They may need special help to readjust, and particularly to re-establish the love and trust that has been lost. Partners have to learn to become re-involved with the drinker in non-drinking activities, but without depriving themselves in any way.

Working with Particular Population Groups

Traditionally, alcohol services have been directed at young and middle-aged men, so specific comment must be made on the needs of other groups.

As alcohol-related problems have increased among men so they have among women, and possibly at an even faster rate. However, there have been relatively few empirical studies on the treatment of female heavy drinkers. The little evidence available suggests that there is not much difference in the outcome of treatment between male and female problem drinkers. However, two points should be noted (39,302). First, women are more likely than men to attribute the onset of their problem to a particular stressful or traumatic event. Second, it does appear that women are more susceptible to the adverse effects of alcohol than men, for which reason lower levels of "safe" consumption are recommended for them.

The home situation is important, and treatment is likely to be more successful in women with a supportive spouse. Unfortunately in about half the cases where a woman is drinking to excess, the partner or husband is doing the same and her drinking may be very much related to his. It is important therefore to try and see both together at some time.

There is little evidence either to substantiate or to refute the notion that women need separate facilities or different kinds of treatment (303).

128

However, there is evidence that women underuse alcohol treatment services, are less likely to take the initiative to get help, and have more family, financial and social difficulties in entering treatment *(304)*. Since women are more likely than men to consult primary health care physicians with a variety of complaints including anxiety and depression, since they sometimes use alcohol to cope with these complaints, and since the abuse of alcohol and the use of prescribed drugs such as the benzodiazepines appear to be associated in women, primary health care staff would seem well placed to detect and respond to drinking problems in women *(305)*.

Between a quarter and a third of the children of families in which one parent is a problem drinker will go the same way themselves. Furthermore, there is a high rate of emotional disturbance in families with problem drinkers, especially if physical violence occurs. It is important, therefore, for the therapist to see the children, assess them and find out how they feel about what is going on in the family; the children themselves may need psychological assistance and in severe cases should be helped to understand what is happening and how they can cope with it. Schools, school counselling services, youth services, and bodies such as Al-Ateen (an association for the teenage children of problem drinkers, linked to Al-Anon and Alcoholics Anonymous) can all help. Small children may be at risk of abuse or neglect from heavily drinking parents. However, it is important not to stigmatize a parent, and especially not a mother, simply on account of the drinking.

Child drinkers sometimes come into contact with alcohol services at a very early age. They can suffer all sorts of harm due to alcohol and may be abusing any of a wide range of legal and/or illicit drugs as well. Teenagers with drinking problems seldom present themselves to care agencies, and there has been very little research into the treatment of alcohol problems in the young. The same principles probably apply, however, as to adults. The young do benefit from a positive approach to treatment; a discussion of healthy drinking choices may be more constructive than the suggestion that only heavy drinking is bad.

The elderly
Increasing attention is now being given to the fact that elderly people have at least their fair share, if not more, of drinking problems *(306–308)* although very little research has actually been done on alcohol consumption in this group. It is easy to miss the symptoms of heavy drinking among signs of the physical deterioration, intellectual decline and social isolation to which the elderly are prone.

Self-neglect, falls, burns, failure to take medication correctly, forgetfulness, confusion and hypothermia should all alert primary health care staff to possible alcohol problems. It is particularly important to make sure that older people eat well, get enough vitamins, and avoid taking alcohol together with other drugs.

129

Minority groups

Europe has many ethnic minorities, and there is no reason to think that they are immune from alcohol problems; indeed, the contrary is true according to treatment agencies and community workers.

People from minority groups should be treated in the same way as anyone else, except that the therapist should be alert to the influence of cultural factors and differences of attitude and behaviour. Drinking norms may differ, and a level of drinking that would not be a problem in a majority group may be so in a minority group, or vice versa. It may also be easier (or more difficult) to involve a close family member in the patient's treatment. Family attitudes to heavy drinking, violence, separation and divorce can be very different from one ethnic group to another.

The single homeless drinker

Although such a small minority of problem drinkers fall into this group, they are the most visible and readily identified *(308)*. They clearly present special problems, and their short-term prognosis is not favourable. However, rehabilitation is a realistic aim for most single homeless drinkers, and the doctor needs to maintain a positive attitude and give skilful counselling. Doctors should also know about and enlist the help of agencies that have particular experience in this field.

Many countries have tried alternatives to prison as a way of dealing with single homeless drinkers. Since 1956, Poland has had sobering-up stations where a drunk brought in by a police officer can be examined by a doctor, bathed and put to bed. The person leaves the next morning, and only if he or she is readmitted is further action taken.

In Scotland a controlled trial was set up to evaluate a detoxification project. Fifty-two patients were given a yellow card, which meant that whenever they were picked up by the police they were taken to the detoxification centre, whereas the 49 controls were dealt with in the usual way. The results showed that a detoxification centre was certainly effective, although there were many problems. At the end of the trial the regularly detoxified patients were found to have better accommodation and drinking habits than the controls, but only the former improvement was of statistical significance. Some attempt was made to cost the exercise. The detoxified patients cost the taxpayer about 20% more during the experimental year than in the year before they were enrolled in the trial *(309)*.

Doctors

In many countries medical practitioners have higher death rates from cirrhosis than the general population, and alcohol is one of the most common causes of a doctor's inability to practise competently. A considerable proportion of doctors with alcohol problems also use other drugs. Some begin drinking after using other drugs, but more commonly the hung-over doctor experiments with other drugs and then becomes dependent on them as well.

The main problem for drinking doctors is lack of help from their colleagues. "For the doctor-alcoholic, the familiar history is therefore of a period of very dangerous drinking during which his colleagues have turned a blind eye, with the story developing to a crisis which is met with misunderstanding and rejection" (310).

Sadly, doctors with alcohol problems only rarely seek help of their own accord, and even then they are concerned not so much about their consumption as about its adverse consequences. Family, friends and colleagues must make it clear to any doctor who is drinking excessively that they are worried about it; not to do so merely hastens the day when someone will have to act, perhaps dramatically and publicly, because of a crisis. Once a doctor has come forward for help, treatment is much the same as for anyone else, but the outcome can be very poor indeed if there has been too much delay in seeking help (311).

Other Potential Resources

Occupational health services
As already mentioned in Chapter 4, an alcohol service at the workplace may be a good idea for several reasons (312). First, most people with alcohol problems are employed, and the problems often become apparent at work; second, certain occupations are associated with an increased prevalence of alcohol problems; third, the cost of alcohol abuse to employers is considerable; and fourth, people whose livelihood is at stake are likely to be strongly motivated to overcome their problems.

Occupational health policies on alcohol have two components. One concerns alcohol consumption at work during working hours; the other is part of the employer's policy on sickness generally. Where a work policy can be agreed, it will probably aim at prevention, identification of problems, and referral or counselling. The policy must apply to all workers and be in written form. It should be easily visible, so that everybody in the company knows that it exists. The stated objectives must be to help problem drinkers in the interests of health and safety at work. The employer's intentions regarding confidentiality, job security, sickness benefit, pension rights and disciplinary procedures must be clearly specified.

Most programmes consist mainly of the detection of problem drinkers, who are then referred to the occupational physician.

Student health services
Heavy drinking and related damage are common among students (313), and student health centre staff need to be aware that it can be an important factor in many consultations. Universities and colleges should consider

controlling both the availability and consumption of alcohol on their premises. Health education material can be circulated to students, and those responsible for the student health service should look into the example set by teaching staff and older students to younger ones.

Police surgeons
Police surgeons are called upon to distinguish between the effects of alcohol and medical conditions, particularly trauma in people detained by the police, and perform statutory duties connected with the laws on drinking-and-driving, drunkenness in public places, and so on. They can also play a preventive role by alerting primary health care staff to people with drinking-and-driving problems and by talking to them about alcohol as a cause of various social problems.

Prison services
Alcohol-related problems are very common among prisoners *(107)*, some of whom are in prison because of their drinking. The latter are often so-called "habitual drunken offenders", who pass in and out of prison, usually serving short sentences. All that prison has to offer them is detoxification, a month or so without drink, a roof over their heads and a reasonable diet. It has been agreed for more than a century that prison is not the place for them, but in many countries attempts to find better solutions seem to have failed.

Other prisoners also have many alcohol problems: when comparisons can be made, such problems seem to be commoner on the inside than outside. By definition, many prisons are alcohol-free, so that the success of counselling or other therapy in prison is hard to gauge until the prisoner is released into the real world of temptation, where alcohol is available and people are drinking all around. However, useful work could be done in prison by making an assessment, as outlined earlier (p. 108). Workshops can be run for heavy drinkers by probation officers, alcohol counsellors, or other specialists who visit the prison.

Organic and Other Problems

Liver disease
Where liver disease is diagnosed, initial total abstinence is essential and the patient must take a good diet and supplementary vitamins, especially the B complex. If liver disease is recognized early enough and adequately treated, the improvement can be rapid and striking; indeed, in the absence of other diagnostic pointers, such an improvement is a powerful confirmation that the liver was damaged by alcohol.

Most people who have had an adverse hepatic reaction to alcohol should abstain for a prolonged period. For some, however, a return to modest consumption may be acceptable after 3–6 months. If a liver biopsy has been performed, this will help in the decision *(314)*.

People with acute alcoholic hepatitis often deteriorate in hospital at the beginning; it may take 1–6 months before they get any better and up to a half may die. The prognosis for alcoholic cirrhosis, however, is much better than for other forms of the disease, although success depends on the patient stopping drinking. In one study, 69% of those who abstained were alive after five years, compared to only 34% of those who continued to drink *(315)*.

Neurological damage
The clinical and pathological evidence suggests that nutritional deficiency is a major factor in most neurological disease associated with heavy alcohol consumption *(113)*. The relationship between Wernicke's encephalopathy and thiamine deficiency is well established, and signs of the former respond rapidly to administration of the latter. The relationship between thiamine deficiency and Korsakoff's psychosis is less clear. Thiamine reduces symptoms of apathy and improves the ability to concentrate, whereas memory defect may recover slowly, incompletely, or not at all.

Other organic problems
The medical control of certain other problems, such as diabetes and high blood pressure, will improve with a reduction of alcohol intake. Many of the less serious symptoms — such as anxiety, sleeplessness, sickness and bowel disturbance — get better when the patient cuts down; there is little point, in fact, in treating any of them until a reduction in intake has been shown not to help. Indeed, it may be dangerous to treat many of the symptoms of alcohol consumption. It is too easy to replace one drug (alcohol) with another (a tranquillizer).

Violence
Police may be reluctant to involve themselves in domestic disputes unless serious violence occurs. This is usually because once the crisis is over the spouse (usually the wife) is often reluctant to proceed with charges against a husband who by this time is full of promises that it will not happen again. Many wives, rather than calling the police, call the doctor in the hope that the husband can be taken forcibly into hospital or given medication to calm him down. If such a request is made, the doctor should ascertain the exact circumstances of any threats, and also whether the situation has occurred before and with what results. He or she will then have to weigh up the risks of aggravating the trouble, or of becoming personally involved in any violence. If the doctor is satisfied that no serious risk of violence exists, nor any serious medical condition, the caller should be advised to allow the drinker to sleep off the effects. If

serious risk is involved, either those in the vicinity should remove themselves or, if they are unable to, the police should be called.

Suicide

Although the threat of suicide is real (and there is a high suicide rate among heavy drinkers) it is much less frequent in those who live with their families. In cases of a suicide threat, it is better to visit the patient. The doctor should first assess whether the drinker has injured himself or herself at all, and if so should arrange appropriate treatment. Usually the threat of suicide rapidly recedes as the patient sobers up, but the patient should continue to be observed, preferably by members of the family. If there is a history of previous suicide attempts, or the patient is suffering from delirium tremens or withdrawal, hospital admission is needed.

Intoxication

It is pointless to try to discuss alcohol problems with a person who is drunk. He or she needs to sober up and if necessary be helped to cover up the withdrawal symptoms.

There can be real danger from acute intoxication, and if there is any doubt the patient should be admitted to hospital. Blood alcohol concentrations above 400 mg per 100 ml carry for most people a serious risk of coma and death from respiratory depression or aspiration of vomit. A breathalyser can be very useful in such cases.

Intoxication may lead to, but also be aggravated or mimicked by, a number of important conditions:

— cerebral injury, concussion, or extradural or subdural haemor-rhage;

— hypoglycaemia, mainly in malnourished drinkers; and

— opportunistic infection, especially meningitis.

It may also lead to, or be aggravated or mimicked by, the use of other drugs.

Referral

The majority of heavy drinkers and people with alcohol problems can be helped by support from members of the primary health care team and from their families. However, there are some drinkers, particularly those who have severe problems, who lack a supportive family, who have a severe psychological problem, or in whose case treatment has previously failed, who will need to be referred. After referral it is important to maintain a relationship with the patient, and to give the patient another appointment to discuss the result, otherwise the referral may be seen as a rejection.

The resources available for referral have already been mentioned in Chapter 4, the optimum being the following.

Voluntary counselling services
In some places voluntary agencies exist that coordinate the services available to heavy drinkers and provide counselling and advice for them and their families. Some such agencies help people who use any of a wide range of drugs, including alcohol and tranquillizers. Voluntary agencies usually accept clients who walk in off the street, as well as those referred to them from elsewhere.

Community-based alcohol services
Community-based alcohol services consisting of multidisciplinary teams made up of social workers, probation officers, psychiatric nurses, counsellors, psychologists and others are sometimes attached or at least linked to alcohol treatment units.

Alcoholics Anonymous
Alcoholics Anonymous is a supportive self-help group. It asks its members to acknowledge that they are alcoholic, and that abstinence is the only way to recovery. Some people are put off by Alcoholics Anonymous' quasi-religious undertones, but there is actually no requirement for members to worship or to believe. It may be necessary to shop around before finding a group that suits a particular personality. Professional staff can get to know a few Alcoholics Anonymous members personally, and refer their patients to them. Al-Anon and Al-Ateen provide support for the spouses and teenage children of problem drinkers.

Alcohol treatment units
Alcohol treatment units are sometimes associated with psychiatric units, have facilities for detoxification, and offer a range of treatments. Some use a psychoanalytical approach with the emphasis on group work, others a more behaviourist approach. Some operate mostly in a psychiatric hospital, others run more of their services in the community. Some run detoxification and treatment as an integrated service, while others keep the detoxification period separate from the treatment programme. It may be, therefore, that the service offered will not suit the needs of some patients, which can create problems for primary health care staff. Patients who admit a problem but do not consider that it is psychiatric, or who do not like their first experience of group therapy, may be helped more successfully by a voluntary service, if available.

Hostels
Therapeutic hostels and "dry" or "half-way" houses are provided by some municipal and health authorities, and by voluntary agencies. They cater principally but not exclusively for homeless problem drinkers, and also provide temporary shelter for problem drinkers discharged from hospital and habitual drunken offenders discharged from prison.

8

Education, training
and research

Education and Training

A number of researchers have enquired into the educational needs of those working in primary health care *(316–319)*. Anderson *(317)* studied primary health care physicians in England, using the Alcohol and Alcohol Problems Perception Questionnaire *(320)* to investigate their attitudes to working with drinkers (Table 32). Whereas 93% of the doctors studied felt that they had a legitimate right to work with drinkers, only 44% felt capable of doing so and only 39% were motivated to do so. Only 29% were satisfied with the way in which they worked with drinkers, and less than 1 in 10 obtained job satisfaction from the work.

These studies have highlighted the relationship between doctors' attitudes to working with drinkers and their experience: the greater the experience, the more positive the attitude. The studies also suggest a number of ways of overcoming the difficulties that practitioners experience in dealing with alcohol-related problems.

The first need is for better education and training. Despite the changes that have been made to accommodate an introduction to and training for general practice, medical education still does not prepare doctors adequately for the kinds of problem presented to them in general practice. The second need is for support services. The work of Shaw and his colleagues *(190)* has shown that acquiring experience of dealing with drinking problems in a supportive environment is a crucial element in securing professional commitment to the detection and management of alcohol problems.

The third need is for coordination and cooperation. It remains likely that the development of community alcohol teams as recommended by Shaw et al. is potentially the most effective approach to securing general practitioners' commitment to detecting and managing alcohol problems. A willingness on the part of specialists to work within general practice, rather than wait for general practitioners and patients to come to them,

Table 32. Attitude questionnaire

Below are a series of statements about working with drinkers. Please indicate how much you agree or disagree with each statement by ringing the appropriate number. The term drinker is used to refer to a person with alcohol-related problems.

	Strongly agree	Quite strongly agree	Agree	Neither agree nor disagree	Disagree	Quite strongly disagree	Strongly disagree
1. I feel I know enough about the causes of drinking problems to carry out my role when working with drinkers.	7	6	5	4	3	2	1
2. I feel I can appropriately advise my patients about drinking and its effects.	7	6	5	4	3	2	1
3. I feel I have the right to ask patients questions about their drinking when necessary.	7	6	5	4	3	2	1
4. I feel that my patients believe I have the right to ask them questions about drinking when necessary.	7	6	5	4	3	2	1
5. I want to work with drinkers.	7	6	5	4	3	2	1
6. All in all I am inclined to feel I am a failure with drinkers.	7	6	5	4	3	2	1
7. I feel I do not have much to be proud of when working with drinkers.	7	6	5	4	3	2	1
8. Pessimism is the most realistic attitude to take towards drinkers.	7	6	5	4	3	2	1
9. In general, it is rewarding to work with drinkers.	7	6	5	4	3	2	1
10. In general, I like drinkers.	7	6	5	4	3	2	1

Source: Anderson & Clement (321).

and the provision of opportunities for doctors to meet colleagues in their own and related professions, could also go some way towards encouraging general practitioners to work with drink problems.

The fourth and last need is for a change in public attitudes. Educational change and the provision of a supportive environment can at best be only a partial answer to physicians' difficulties; at worst, by emphasizing the medical response to alcohol problems, they divert attention away from the importance of political and social factors. It is unrealistic to expect general practitioners to respond enthusiastically to the task of detecting and managing alcohol problems while political and economic interests sustain existing public beliefs and attitudes towards drinking; this only makes it difficult for doctors and patients alike to acknowledge the existence of the alcohol problem.

It is an open question as to who are the most appropriate educators of primary health care physicians — other doctors or specialists. Some departments pay general practitioners to come in for one or more sessions at which they help specialists and generalists work together to improve the management of conditions such as asthma or recurrent chest pain *(322)*. This approach is ideal for alcohol problems: it brings generalist and specialist together, but ensures that learning and management remain focused on primary health care.

Undergraduates
Although many medical schools arrange some formal teaching on alcohol, very few use an integrated multidisciplinary approach *(323)*. Most teaching is ad hoc and given by psychiatrists, physicians, pharmacologists, general practitioners and pathologists. Only occasionally are behavioural scientists or psychologists involved. The teaching is therefore predominantly medical, so that medical students are likely to adopt attitudes to alcohol that are curative and palliative, rather than preventive and promotive.

Teaching on alcohol should not only be concerned with facts and skills, but should also offer students the opportunity to explore their own attitudes and behaviour towards alcohol *(324)*. This would have two benefits: first, it would help students think about their own use of alcohol both now and in the future; and second, it would help them understand the relationship between their own attitudes and behaviour and their responsibilities towards their patients.

Departments of general practice or of community and family medicine should be responsible for alcohol education programmes in the medical school. These programmes would then be a natural extension of the multidisciplinary work already being done, emphasizing epidemiology and sociology and including concepts that narrow the gap between the normal and the abnormal. They would help students understand the variability of lifestyle and how it relates to the natural history of, for

139

example, raised blood pressure, overweight and dependence on cigarettes. All three conditions may be helped by interventions at any stage, or they may resolve themselves spontaneously. Once involved in care, the primary health physician becomes part of a process that may be lifelong and embrace the patient, the family and other professional and lay groups and individuals. The problems posed by alcohol are excellent material for multidisciplinary teaching, which should stress that a reduction in alcohol problems would go a long way towards eliminating the other conditions mentioned above *(325–327)*.

Heavy drinkers seeking help have many choices: they can go to primary health care physicians, psychiatrists, community alcohol teams, psychologists, social workers, probation officers and so on. If they choose to see a doctor it is probable, and usually desirable, that other disciplines will be involved, so these disciplines should also be involved in medical teaching *(328)*. Multidisciplinary workshops, where students do group work and explore their own attitudes to alcohol and to people with alcohol-related problems, can be used to illustrate more general questions.

Examinations have a powerful influence on the direction of medical students' work and the effort they put into it. If students are to appreciate the value of teaching on alcohol, then they should be examined on it and assessed during the course itself *(328)*.

Higher professional training
There is also considerable scope for alcohol education in higher professional training *(329)*. Most vocational training schemes give time to counselling and consulting skills. A number of training manuals and attitude questionnaires (Table 32) are available *(6,36,321)*.

Continuing education
The main objective of continuing education is to equip the doctor with new knowledge and new skills as they emerge during the doctor's professional life, although this "re-tooling" is only part of the process *(322)*. Another objective is to improve the quality of clinical medicine by ensuring that the knowledge and skills thus acquired are also properly applied. For some doctors this requires a renewal or renaissance of the enthusiasm and commitment they felt during the first few years in practice. Often the first 5 or even 10 years of a doctor's working life are full of interest, but after that they have solved many of the organizational problems and become familiar with the most common dilemmas. There then stretches out before them a plateau, another 25 or 30 years of professional life, doing much the same kind of thing. Only a few will manage to retain their freshness and enthusiasm and continue to seek new ways to improve the quality of the service they provide.

Commitment to the improvement of quality is influenced by many variables and its distribution, like that of blood pressure, would probably prove to be Gaussian if there were an easy way of measuring it. The greatest number — the hump of the curve — are keen to improve quality, but need practical assistance and not vague exhortations before they can translate good intentions into better practice. Furthermore, the method of assistance must be acceptable to most doctors and not just to a few: the impact on public health would be greater if the majority were to improve their effectiveness by 5% than if the keenest were to improve their already excellent service by 10% or the worst by 200%.

The principles of effective continuing medical education have been listed as follows *(330,331)*:

— continuing education should be based on the doctor's own work as well as on research findings;

— the doctor should be helped to assess his or her work and to compare it with that of others;

— where teamwork is necessary for good quality care, the whole team should be involved;

— continuing education programmes should be developed in collaboration with doctors, rather than being imposed on them;

— the views of patients should be incorporated;

— continuing education should help the physician not only to acquire new knowledge and skills, but also to change the way he or she works;

— it must be based on the assumption that doctors are busy, but that the great majority would like to improve the quality of care they provide; and finally

— continuing education should be enjoyable.

The seminar or lecture is a common medium for continuing medical education. Although the transmission of information by itself does not necessarily improve performance, seminars planned with a specific objective and organized for doctors who are providing a service can be effective. In a hypertension education project, it was found that the patients of doctors who had attended a single tutorial achieved lower blood pressures than did the patients of doctors in a control group *(332)*. It is often practical difficulties that prevent interested doctors from attending seminars, and many are attended only by a proportion of those who could benefit from them. The coverage can be increased by complementing the seminar with a written summary or locally produced newsletter that sets out the consensus reached.

Although the most effective learning takes place in a group, well designed material can be used for study at home *(333,334)*. This type of studying is done in the physician's spare time. There are few systems, in

141

fact, that provide physicians with information at the time when they would be most likely to learn from it, that is to say when they are faced with a patient whose difficulty could be satisfactorily solved *(335–337)*.

Referral of the patient to a specialist (and the specialist's reply) affords an important opportunity for continuing education. Doctors can be taught how to use these "teachable moments", and to exploit the information at their disposal in the form of computer data bases, for example. They should also know about telephone hotlines and the other expert services, medical and non-medical, that they and their patients can use.

Doctors need information not only about disease but also about their own performance, and how it compares either with the criteria set out in protocols or with their peers' performance. The fact of informing a doctor that he or she is performing differently from others almost always has an effect by itself, but that effect will usually be to encourage regression to the mean, unless the performance can be compared with what is generally considered to be good practice. Furthermore, the information is even more likely to have an effect if the doctor concerned has actually been involved in defining what constitutes good practice.

Reaching agreement on what constitutes good practice and providing feedback requires a more systematic approach to medical care than exists at present. Protocols, guidelines and algorithms developed as care becomes more systematic are effective, but must be used with caution: their effectiveness is probably due as much to the process of developing them as to the guidelines themselves. Some researchers have found guidelines produced by experts to be effective, but in other cases their strength seems to derive not only from their basis in scientific evidence but also from the involvement of those whose behaviour is to be modified by the guidelines.

Information and feedback are more likely to be effective if presented personally and not by a computer printout. In some systems "educational influentials" (doctors respected by their colleagues) are used; in others a nurse or a pharmacist. Physicians or teams working in isolation are visited by someone competent and acceptable, who brings them information about their own performance and how it compares with what they or their peers accept as good practice. These "facilitators of change" also bring practical offers of assistance, which make a welcome change from vague exhortations by distant authorities.

A facilitator model has been described in which three general practices in the United Kingdom were provided with low-cost, low-technology support from a facilitator, and compared with control practices to see how often they found major risk factors for cardiovascular disease in middle-aged patients *(280,338)*. Patients who consulted general practitioners in the intervention group were recruited to make an appointment with the practice nurse for a health check, and the outcome of this was compared with the outcome of ordinary consultations in the

142

control practices. Intervention practices were helped by the facilitator to develop the nurse's role.

During the study, the intervention practices recorded twice as much high blood pressure, four times as much smoking and five times as much overweight as the control practices. This model is now being applied to screening for alcohol consumption and management of alcohol-related problems in primary health care.

Research Issues

Earlier chapters have pointed to some of the research issues in the prevention and management of alcohol problems in primary health care. There have been three reviews of the international issues *(5,339,340)*, and more recently the *British journal of addiction* has devoted a series of articles to research being done in the European countries *(341–352)*.

Health promotion
Chapter 4 referred to the WHO Healthy Cities initiative and to collaboration with the departments responsible for recreational facilities in municipalities. Further process and outcome evaluation work is required on the various projects of this type; this research should itself have a health promotional effect because local communities will be involved in planning and doing the research and applying its findings.

Policy development and implementation
More research is also needed on local alcohol policy development and implementation (Chapter 5), and especially on ways of encouraging interorganizational collaboration, producing policy process manuals and evaluating policy outcome.

Self-help
Chapter 4 mentioned research into the effectiveness of self-help manuals in helping problem drinkers recruited through articles in newspapers and magazines *(348)*. Further work is now being done in this area, in particular in order to examine more closely the validity of some of the previous findings (especially with respect to the outcome for those with relatively more serious problems), and to assess the added effectiveness of some degree of telephone contact in enabling low-dependence problem drinkers to reduce their drinking *(348)*.

Effectiveness of primary health care interventions
Chapter 7 described some of the primary health care intervention studies undertaken recently. There have been four such studies in the United Kingdom and two in Scandinavia, and others are planned elsewhere in Europe. More work is needed on the most effective components of simple intervention, and on the role of nurses as opposed to doctors in

giving advice to patients to cut down on their drinking. In Scotland, a revised DRAMS scheme is being developed, based on Prochaska and di Clemente's model of the change process and incorporating some of the lessons learned from previous research *(348)*. New materials are also needed for use in primary health care. Both the Netherlands and the United Kingdom have developed primary health care intervention packs consisting of instructional booklets for primary health care staff, and small self-help booklets for patients. Their acceptability and effectiveness need to be further evaluated.

Educational methods
Reference has been made earlier in this chapter to studies of the effectiveness of a number of different techniques for continuing education, including seminars, self-study, using the teachable moment, feedback, development of a system of medical care, and facilitators for change. Many of these evaluation methods have been used in other areas of health care, for example in medical drug therapy, the management of rheumatoid arthritis and the management of pulmonary disease and hypertension. There is now scope for applying the findings of this research to the education of primary health care staff on the subject of alcohol. A current research project in the United Kingdom is in fact testing the effectiveness of a facilitator for change in the field of alcohol and primary health care. The study takes the form of a randomized controlled trial, in which 10 primary health care group practices receive visits from a facilitator. The facilitator advises the practices on setting up systems for screening for individual patients' alcohol consumption and for teaching the staff simple counselling skills so that they can give advice to heavy drinkers on how to cut down. The facilitator also brings information to the practices about their own performance in these areas and how it compares with what they and their peers accept as good practice. The input in the 10 study practices is being compared with no input in 10 control practices.

Efficiency, effectiveness and rational planning
Chapter 4 emphasized the need to determine all the resources available to a community for preventing and managing alcohol problems, and touched on issues of efficiency, effectiveness and rational planning. Further work is required on defining the needs of local populations and improving the information base so more rational decisions can be made about issues of effectiveness and efficiency.

Marketing of research findings
An organization is needed that can act as a clearing-house and maintain a data base of current activities along the lines of the Alcohol Research Group at the University of Edinburgh with its Register of United Kingdom Alcohol Research *(353)*. There should also be a system for

"marketing" research findings and translating them into clinical practice. As regards continuing medical education particularly, more work needs to be done on relevant research whose findings are then applied promptly for the benefit of patients.

References

1. WHO Technical Report Series No. 650, 1980 (*Problems related to alcohol consumption*: report of a WHO Expert Committee).
2. **Walsh, D.** *Alcohol-related medicosocial problems and their prevention.* Copenhagen, WHO Regional Office for Europe, 1982 (Public Health in Europe No. 17).
3. **Ritson, E.B.** *Community response to alcohol-related problems. Review of an international study.* Geneva, World Health Organization, 1985 (Public Health Papers No. 85).
4. **Rootman, I. & Hughes, P.H.** *Drug-abuse reporting systems.* Geneva, World Health Organization, 1980 (WHO Offset Publication No. 55).
5. **Rootman, I. & Moser, J.** *Guidelines for investigating alcohol problems and developing appropriate responses.* Geneva, World Health Organization, 1984 (WHO Offset Publication No. 81).
6. *Drug dependence and alcohol-related problems. A manual for community health workers, with guidelines for trainers.* Geneva, World Health Organization, 1986.
7. *Treatment and rehabilitation programmes in alcohol abuse.* Copenhagen, WHO Regional Office for Europe, 1986 (unpublished document ICP/ADA 993/s01).
8. *The respective roles of primary health care and specialized services in the development and implementation of programmes for problem drinkers.* Copenhagen, WHO Regional Office for Europe, 1987 (unpublished document ICP/ADA 010).
9. *Working group on implementation and evaluation of programmes for problem drinking*: summary report. Copenhagen, WHO Regional Office for Europe, 1987 (unpublished document EUR/ICP/ADA 031(S)).
10. *International statistics on alcoholic beverages, 1950–1972.* Helsinki, Finnish Foundation for Alcohol Studies, 1977, Vol. 27.

11. **Österberg, E.** *Recorded consumption: Finland 1959–1975.* Helsinki, Social Research Institute of Alcohol Studies, 1979 (Report No. 125).

12. **The Brewers' Society.** *International statistical handbook.* London, Brewing Publications, 1983.

13. **The Brewers' Society.** *Statistical handbook.* London, Brewing Publications, 1985.

14. *Hoeveel alkoholhoudende dranken vorden er in wereld gedronken?* [How much alcohol is drunk in the world?] Schiedam, Produktschap voor Gedistilleerde Dranken, 1986.

15. **Powell, M.** Alcohol data in the European Community. *British journal of addiction,* **82**: 559–566 (1987).

16. **Spring J.A. & Buss, D.H.** Three centuries of alcohol in the British diet. *Nature,* **270**: 567–572 (1977).

17. **Mäkelä, K.** *Unrecorded consumption of alcohol in Finland, 1950–1975.* Helsinki, Social Research Institute of Alcohol Studies, 1979 (Report No. 126).

18. **McDonnell, R.** A review of routine Government data collection on alcohol consumption. *Community medicine,* **8**: 206–223 (1986).

19. **Office of Population Censuses and Surveys.** *General household surveys.* London, H.M. Stationery Office, 1975–1982.

20. **Department of Employment.** *Family expenditure surveys.* London, H.M. Stationery Office, 1978–1982.

21. **Wilson, P.** *Drinking in England and Wales.* London, H.M. Stationery Office, 1980.

22. **Knight, I. & Wilson, P.** *Scottish licensing laws.* London, H.M. Stationery Office, 1980.

23. **Breeze, E.** *Differences in drinking patterns between selected regions.* London, H.M. Stationery Office, 1985.

24. **Breeze, E.** *Women and drinking survey.* London, H.M. Stationery Office, 1985.

25. **Davie, R. et al.** *From birth to seven. The second report of the National Child Development Study.* London, National Children's Bureau, 1972.

26. **Knibbe, R.A. et al.** The development of alcohol consumption in the Netherlands: 1958–1981. *British journal of addiction,* **80**: 411–419 (1985).

27. **Pernanen, K.** Validity of survey data on alcohol use. *In:* Gibbons, R.J. et al., ed. *Research advances in alcohol and drug problems.* New York, Wiley, 1974, Vol. I.

28. **Wilson, P.** Improving the methodology of drinking surveys. *Statistician,* **30**: 159–167 (1981).

29. **Duffy, J.C. & Waterton, J.J.** Under-reporting of alcohol consumption in sample surveys: the effect of computer interviewing in fieldwork. *British journal of addiction,* **79**: 303–308 (1984).

30. **Crawford, A.** Bias in a survey of drinking habits. *Alcohol and alcoholism,* **2:** 167–179 (1987).

31. **Romelsjo, A.** *Alcohol consumption and social data in Stockholm, 1984.* Paper presented to the Alcohol Epidemiology Section, ICAA, Dubrovnik, 8–13 June 1986.

32. **Crawford, A.** A comparison of participants and non-participants from a British general population survey of alcohol drinking practices. *Journal of the Market Research Society,* **28:** 291–297 (1986).

33. **Poikolainen, K. & Karkkainen, P.** *Diary gives more accurate information about alcohol consumption than questionnaire.* Paper presented to Alcohol Epidemiology Section, ICAA, Padua, 20–24 June 1983.

34. **Poikolainen, K. & Karkkainen, P.** Nature of questionnaire options affects estimate of alcohol intake. *Journal of studies on alcohol,* **46:** 210–222 (1985).

35. **Robertson, I. et al.** *Psychology and problem drinking.* Leicester, British Psychological Society, 1984.

36. *Alcohol — a balanced view.* London, Royal College of General Practitioners, 1986.

37. **Jessor, R. & Jessor, S.** *Problem behaviour and psychological developments: a longitudinal study of youth.* New York, Academic Press, 1977.

38. **Vuchinich, R. et al.** Alcohol, cognitive labelling and mirth. *Journal of abnormal psychology,* **88:** 641–651 (1979).

39. **Annis, H.M.** Treatment of alcoholic women. *In:* Edwards, G. & Grant, M., ed. *Alcoholism treatment in transition.* London, Croom Helm, 1980.

40. **Jacob, T. & Seilhamer, R.A.** The impact on spouses and how they cope. *In:* Orford, J. & Harwin, J. *Alcohol and the family.* London, Croom Helm, 1982.

41. **Plant, M.A.** *Drinking careers: occupations, drinking habits and drinking problems.* London, Tavistock, 1979.

42. *Alcohol — reducing the harm.* London, Office of Health Economics, 1981.

43. **O'Connor, J.** *The young drinkers.* London, Tavistock, 1978.

44. **Plant, M.A.** Risk factors in employment. *In:* Hore, B.D. & Plant, M.A., ed. *Alcohol problems in employment.* London, Croom Helm, 1981.

45. **Kendell, R. et al.** Effect of economic changes on Scottish drinking habits 1978–1982. *British journal of addiction,* **78:** 365–379 (1983).

46. **Schaefer, J.** Ethnic differences in response to alcohol. *In:* Pickens, R. & Heston, L., ed. *Psychiatric factors in drug abuse.* New York, Grune and Stratton, 1979.

47. **Reinert, R.** The concept of alcoholism as a bad habit. *Bulletin of the Menninger Clinic*, **32**: 35–46 (1968).
48. **Orford, J.** Alcohol problems and the family. *In*: Lishman, J. & Horobin, G., ed. *Approaches to addiction*. London, Kogan Page, 1985.
49. **Vaillant, G.** *The natural history of alcoholism*. London, Harvard University Press, 1983.
50. **Haskey, J.C. et al.** Regional variations in alcohol-related problems within the United Kingdom. *Community medicine*, **5**: 208–209 (1983).
51. **Kilich, S. & Plant, M.A.** Regional variations in levels of alcohol-related problems in Britain. *British journal of addiction*, **76**: 47–62 (1981).
52. **Latcham, R. et al.** Regional variations in British alcohol morbidity rates: a myth uncovered? I. Clinical surveys. *British medical journal*, **289**: 1341–1343 (1984).
53. **Crawford, A. et al.** Regional variations in British alcohol morbidity rates: a myth uncovered? II. General population surveys. *British medical journal*, **289**: 1343–1345 (1984).
54. **Crawford, A. et al.** Self-reported alcohol consumption and adverse consequences of drinking in three areas of Britain: general population surveys. *British journal of addiction*, **80**: 421–428 (1985).
55. **Ledermann, S.** *Alcool, alcoolisme, alcoolisation*. Paris, Presses Universitaires de France, 1956.
56. **Miller, E.H. & Agnew, N.** The Ledermann model of alcohol consumption. *Quarterly journal of studies on alcohol*, **35**: 877–878 (1974).
57. **Duffy, J.** Estimating the proportion of heavy drinkers. *In*: Davies, D.L., ed. *The Ledermann curve*. London, Alcohol Education Centre, 1977.
58. **Skog, O.-J.** On the distribution of alcohol consumption. *In*: Davies, D.L., ed. *The Ledermann curve*. London, Alcohol Education Centre, 1977.
59. **Kreitman, N.** Three themes in the epidemiology of alcoholism. *In*: Edwards, G. & Grant, M., ed. *Alcoholism: new knowledge and new responses*. London, Croom Helm, 1977.
60. **Plant, M.A. & Pirie, F.** Self-reported alcohol consumption and alcohol-related problems: a study in four Scottish towns. *Social psychiatry*, **14**: 65–73 (1979).
61. **Royal College of Psychiatrists.** *Alcohol and alcoholism.* London, Tavistock, 1979.
62. **Österberg, E.** *Indicators of damage and the development of alcohol conditions in Finland during the years 1950–75*. Paper presented at the ISACE Second Working Meeting, Pacific Grove, CA, 1979.

63. Cartwright, A.K.J. et al. The relationships between per capita consumption, drinking patterns and alcohol-related problems in a population sample, 1965–74. Part II: Implications for alcohol control policy. *British journal of addiction*, **73**: 247–258 (1978).

64. Norström, T. The impact of per capita consumption on Swedish cirrhosis mortality. *British journal of addiction*, **82**: 67–75 (1987).

65. Popham, R.E. et al. The prevention of alcoholism: epidemiological studies of the effects of government control measures. *British journal of addiction*, **70**: 125–144 (1975).

66. Havge, R. & Irgens-Jensen, O. The relationship between alcohol consumption, alcohol intoxication and negative consequences of drinking in four Scandinavian countries. *British journal of addiction*, **81**: 513–524 (1986).

67. Skog, O.-S. Trends in alcohol consumption and deaths from diseases. *British journal of addiction*, **81**: 1033–1041 (1986).

68. Skog, O.-J. Trends in alcohol consumption and violent deaths. *British journal of addiction*, **81**: 365–379 (1986).

69. Kendell, R.E. The beneficial consequences of the United Kingdom's declining per capita consumption of alcohol in 1979–1982. *Alcohol and alcoholism*, **19**: 271–276 (1984).

70. Romelsjö, A. & Agren, G. Has mortality related to alcohol decreased in Sweden? *British medical journal*, **291**: 167–170 (1985).

71. Romelsjö, A. Decline in alcohol-related problems in Sweden greatest among young people. *British journal of addiction*, **82**: 1111–1126 (1987).

72. Petersson, B. et al. Risk factors for premature death in middle-aged men. *British medical journal*, **288**: 1264–1268 (1984).

73. McDonnel, R. & Maynard, A. Estimation of life years lost from alcohol-related premature death. *Alcohol and alcoholism*, **20**: 435–443 (1985).

74. Kagan, A. et al. Factors related to stroke incidence in Hawaii Japanese men. *Stroke*, **11**: 15–21 (1980).

75. Kagan, A. et al. Alcohol and cardiovascular disease: the Hawaiian experience. *Circulation*, **64**(Suppl. 3): 27–31 (1981).

76. Kozarevic, D.J. et al. Frequency of alcohol consumption and morbidity and mortality: the Yugoslavia Cardiovascular Disease Study. *Lancet*, **1**: 613–616 (1980).

77. Kozarevic, D.J. et al. Drinking habits and death. *International journal of epidemiology*, **12**: 145–150 (1983).

78. Dyer, A.R. et al. Alcohol consumption and 17-year mortality in the Chicago Western Electric Company Study. *Preventive medicine*, **9**: 78–90 (1980).

79. Dyer, A.R. et al. Alcohol, cardiovascular risk factors and mortality: the Chicago experience. *Circulation*, **64**(Suppl. 3): 20–27 (1981).

80. **Rothman, K.J.** The proportion of cancer attributable to alcohol consumption. *Preventive medicine*, **9**: 174–179 (1980).

81. **Holtermann, S. & Burchell, A.** *The costs of alcohol misuse.* London, Department of Health and Social Security, 1981.

82. **Adelstein, A. & White, G.** Alcoholism and mortality. *Population trends*, **6**: 7–13 (1976).

83. **Marmot, M.G.** Alcohol and coronary heart disease. *International journal of epidemiology*, **13**: 160–167 (1984).

84. **Klatsky, A.L. et al.** Alcohol use and cardiovascular disease: the Kaiser-Permanente experience. *Circulation*, **64**(Suppl. 3): 32–41 (1981).

85. **McDonnel, R. & Maynard, A.** The costs of alcohol misuse. *British journal of addiction*, **80**: 27–35 (1985).

86. **McDonnel, R. & Maynard, A.** Counting the cost of alcohol: gaps in the epidemiological knowledge. *Community medicine*, **7**: 4–17 (1985).

87. **Jariwalla, A.G. et al.** Alcohol and acute general medical admissions to hospital. *Health trends*, **11**: 95–97 (1979).

88. **Jarman, C.M.B. & Kellett, J.M.** Alcoholism in the general hospital. *British medical journal*, **2**: 469–472 (1979).

89. **Quinn, M. & Johnstone, R.** Alcohol problems in acute male medical admissions. *Health bulletin of the Scottish Home and Health Department*, **34**: 253 (1976).

90. **Lennox, I.M. & Tait, C.M.** Blood alcohol levels in acute female medical admissions. *Health bulletin of the Scottish Home and Health Department*, **37**: 127–129 (1979).

91. **Northcote, R.J. et al.** Changing pattern of alcohol abuse in female acute medical admissions. *British medical journal*, **286**: 1702 (1983).

92. **Jellinek, E.M.** Phases of alcohol addiction. *Quarterly journal of studies on alcohol*, **13**: 673–684 (1952).

93. **Edwards, G. & Gross, M.M.** Alcohol dependence: provisional description of a clinical syndrome. *British medical journal*, **1**: 1058–1061 (1976).

94. **Edwards, G. et al., ed.** *Alcohol-related disabilities.* Geneva, World Health Organization, 1977 (WHO Offset Publications No. 32).

95. **Freeman, S.D.A.** *Violence in the home.* Farnborough, Saxon House, 1979.

96. **Cork, R.M.** *The forgotten children: a study of children with alcoholic parents.* Toronto, Addiction Research Foundation, 1969.

97. **Wilson, C. & Orford, J.** Children of alcoholics: report of a preliminary study and comments on the literature. *Journal of studies on alcohol*, **39**: 121–142 (1978).

98. **El-Guebaly, N. & Offored, D.** The offspring of alcoholics: a critical review. *American journal of psychiatry*, **134**: 357–365 (1977).
99. **Bailey, M. et al.** Outcomes of alcoholic marriages: endurance, termination or recovery. *Quarterly journal of studies on alcohol*, **23**: 610–623 (1962).
100. **Nylander, I.** Children of alcoholic fathers. *Acta paediatrica scandinavica*, **49**(Suppl. 121) (1960).
101. **Orme, T.C. & Rimmer, H.** Alcohol and child abuse: a review. *Journal of studies on alcohol*, **42**: 273–287 (1981).
102. **Karlsson, J.** Mental characteristics of families with alcoholism in Iceland. *Hereditas*, **102**: 185–188 (1985).
103. **Rydelius, P.** Children of alcoholic fathers: their social adjustment and their health status over 20 years. *Acta paediatrica scandinavica*, Suppl. 286, pp. 10–85 (1981).
104. **Velleman, R. & Orford, J.** Intergenerational transmission of alcohol problems: hypotheses to be tested. *In*: Krasner, N. et al., ed. *Alcohol-related problems: room for manoeuvre*. Chichester, Wiley, 1984.
105. **Winton, M. et al.** Effects of unemployment on drinking behaviour: a review of the relevant evidence. *International journal of the addictions*, **21**: 1261–1283 (1986).
106. **Iversen, L. & Klausen, H.** *Lukningen af Nordhavnsvaerftet* [The closure of Nordhavn Wharf]. Copenhagen, University of Copenhagen, Institute for Social Medicine, 1981 (Publication No. 13).
107. **Smith, R.** Prison health care. London, *British medical journal*, 1984.
108. **Jeffs, B. & Saunders, W.** Minimising alcohol-related offences by enforcement of existing licensing legislation. *British journal of addiction*, **78**: 67–77 (1983).
109. **Gillies, H.** Homicide in the West of Scotland. *British journal of psychiatry*, **128**: 105 (1976).
110. **Borkenstein, R.F. et al.** *The role of the drinking driver in traffic accidents*. Bloomingham, Indiana, Department of Police Administration, Indiana University, 1964.
111. **Dunbar, J. et al.** Are problem drinkers dangerous drivers? An investigation of arrest for drinking and driving, serum γ-glutamyltranspeptidase activities, blood alcohol concentrations, and road traffic accidents: the Tayside safe driving project. *British medical journal*, **290**: 827–830 (1985).
112. **Pikkarainen, J. & Pertilla, A.** *Drinking and driving in Finland. Proceedings of the Tenth Congress of the International Association for Accident and Traffic Medicine*. Tokyo, Japanese Council of Traffic Science, 1985.
113. **Thomson, A.D. & Ron, M.A.** Alcohol-related brain damage. *British medical bulletin*, **38**: 87–94 (1982).

114. **Robertson, I.** Does moderate drinking cause mental impairment? *British medical journal*, **289**: 711–712 (1984).
115. **Morgan, M.** Alcohol and nutrition. *British medical bulletin*, **38**: 21–129 (1982).
116. **Chanarin, I.** Haemopoiesis and alcohol. *British medical bulletin*, **38**: 81–86 (1982).
117. **Langman, M.J.S. & Bell, G.D.** Alcohol and the gastrointestinal tract. *British medical bulletin*, **38**: 71–75 (1982).
118. **MacSween, R.M.N.** Alcohol and cancer. *British medical bulletin*, **38**: 31–33 (1982).
119. **Schmidt, W. & Popham, R.E.** The role of drinking and smoking in mortality from cancer and other causes in male alcoholics. *Cancer*, **47**: 1031–1041 (1981).
120. **Osmond, C. et al.** *Trends in cancer mortality 1951–1980*. London, H.M. Stationery Office, 1983 (OPCS Series No. 11).
121. **Lake-Bakaar, G.** Alcohol and the pancreas. *British medical bulletin*, **38**: 57–62 (1982).
122. **Saunders, J.B. et al.** Do women develop alcoholic liver disease more readily than men? *British medical journal*, **282**: 1140–1143 (1981).
123. **Péquignot, G. et al.** Ascitic cirrhosis in relation to alcohol consumption. *International journal of epidemiology*, **7**: 113–120 (1978).
124. **Potter, J.F. et al.** Alcohol and hypertension. *British journal of addiction*, **79**: 365–372 (1984).
125. **Klatsky, A.L. et al.** Alcohol consumption and blood pressure. Kaiser-Permanente multiphasic health examination data. *New England journal of medicine*, **296**: 1194–1200 (1977).
126. **Wilkins, M.R. & Kendall, M.J.** Stroke affecting young men after alcoholic binge. *Lancet*, **291**: 1342 (1985).
127. **Saunders, J.B. et al.** Alcohol-induced hypertension. *Lancet*, **2**: 653–656 (1981).
128. **Alderman, E.L. & Coltort, D.J.** Alcohol and the heart. *British medical bulletin*, **38**: 77–80 (1982).
129. **Thornton, J.R.** Atrial fibrillation in healthy non-alcoholic people after an alcoholic binge. *Lancet*, **2**: 1013–1015 (1984).
130. **Marmot, M.G. et al.** Alcohol and mortality: a U-shaped curve. *Lancet*, **1**: 580–583 (1981).
131. **Harper, C.G. et al.** Brain shrinkage in chronic alcoholics: a pathological study. *British medical journal*, **290**: 501–504 (1985).
132. **Martin, F.C. et al.** Alcoholic muscle disease. *British medical bulletin*, **38**: 53–56 (1982).
133. **Morgan, M. & Pratt, O.E.** Sex, alcohol and the developing foetus. *British medical bulletin*, **38**: 43–52 (1982).

134. **Keilman, P.A.** Alcohol consumption and diabetes mellitus mortality in different countries. *American journal of public health*, **73**: 1316–1317 (1983).

135. **Young, R.J. et al.** Alcohol: another risk factor for diabetic retinopathy? *British medical journal*, **288**: 1035–1037 (1984).

136. **Jones, K.L. et al.** Pattern of malformation in offspring of alcoholic mothers. *Lancet*, **1**: 1267–1271 (1973).

137. **Barrison, I.G. et al.** Adverse effects of alcohol on pregnancy. *British journal of addiction*, **80**: 11–12 (1985).

138. **Harlap, S. & Shiono, P.H.** Alcohol, smoking and the incidence of spontaneous abortions in the first and second trimester. *Lancet*, **2**: 173–176 (1980).

139. **Wright, T.J. et al.** Alcohol consumption, pregnancy and low birth weight. *Lancet*, **1**: 663–665 (1983).

140. **United States Surgeon General.** Advisory on alcohol and pregnancy. *Food and Drug Administration bulletin*, **1**: 9–10 (1981).

141. **Plant, M.** *Women, drinking and pregnancy.* London, Tavistock, 1985.

142. **Schatzkin, A.** Alcohol consumption and breast cancer in the epidemiologic follow-up study of the first national health and nutrition examination survey. *New England journal of medicine*, **316**: 1169–1173 (1987).

143. **Willet, W.C. et al.** Moderate alcohol consumption and the risk of breast cancer. *New England journal of medicine*, **316**: 1174–1180 (1987).

144. **Murray, W.R.** Head injuries and alcohol. *In*: Edwards, G. & Grant, M., ed. *Alcoholism: new knowledge and new responses.* London, Croom Helm, 1977.

145. **Observer and Maxwell, M.A.** A study of absenteeism, accidents and sickness payments in problem drinkers in one industry. *Quarterly journal of studies on alcohol*, **20**: 302–312 (1959).

146. **Tether, P. & Harrison, L.** Alcohol-related fires and drownings. *British journal of addiction*, **81**: 425–431 (1986).

147. **Popham, R.E. et al.** Heavy alcohol consumption and physical health problems. *Research advances in alcohol and drug problems*, **8**: 149–182 (1984).

148. **Turner, T.B. et al.** Measurement of alcohol-related effects in man: chronic effects in relation to levels of alcohol consumption. *Johns Hopkins medical journal*, **141**: 235–248; 273–276 (1977).

149. **Kreitman, N.** Alcohol consumption and the preventive paradox. *British journal of addiction*, **81**: 353–363 (1986).

150. **Klatsky, A.L. et al.** Alcohol and mortality: a ten-year Kaiser-Permanente experience. *Annals of internal medicine*, **95**: 139–145 (1981).

151. **Office of Population Censuses and Surveys.** *General Household Survey 1982.* London, H.M. Stationery Office, 1984.
152. **Office of Population Censuses and Surveys.** *Morbidity statistics from general practice 1971–2.* London, H.M. Stationery Office, 1979 (Studies on Medical and Population Subjects No. 36).
153. **Wilkins, R.H.** *The hidden alcoholic in general practice.* London, Elek Science, 1974.
154. **Gray, J.M.** Four-box health care. Development in a time of zero growth. *Lancet,* **2**: 1185–1186 (1983).
155. **Rush, B.** *A model for estimating required service capacities for addiction treatment programmes in Ontario: executive summary and recommendations for application.* Toronto, Addiction Research Foundation, 1988.
156. **Ruch, B. & Ekdahl, A.** *Treatment services for alcohol and drug abuse in Ontario: results of a provincial survey, 1986.* Toronto, Addiction Research Foundation, 1987.
157. **Giesbrecht, N. & Conroy, G.** Options in developing community action against alcohol problems. *In*: Holder, H.D., ed. Central issues in alcohol abuse prevention: strategies for states and communities. *Advances in substance abuse*, Suppl. 1, pp. 315–335 (1987).
158. **Giesbrecht, N.** *Planning community strategies on alcohol issues: notes from a multi-component prevention initiative.* Toronto, Addiction Research Foundation, 1986.
159. **Thomson, M. & Douglas, R.R.** *A peek into the black box. A policy development model for the resolution of social and health issues in municipal recreation.* Toronto, Addiction Research Foundation, 1983 (ARF Internal Document No. 3).
160. **Thomson, M. et al.** *Implementing a policy to manage alcohol in municipal recreational facilities: influencing participants to play by the rules.* Toronto, Addiction Research Foundation, 1985 (ARF Internal Document No. 54).
161. **Gliksman, L. et al.** *The impact of a promotional campaign on a community's intention to comply with a policy to manage alcohol in its municipally owned recreational facilities.* Toronto, Addiction Research Foundation, 1987 (ARF Internal Document No. 82).
162. **Single, E.** Studies of public drinking: an overview. *In*: Single, E. & Storm, T., ed. *Public drinking and public policy.* Toronto, Addiction Research Foundation, 1985.
163. **Single, E.** The control of public drinking: the impact of the environment on alcohol problems. *In*: Holder, H.D., ed. Control issues in alcohol abuse prevention: strategies for states and communities. *Advances in substance abuse*, Suppl. 7, pp. 219–232 (1987).
164. **Simpson, R. et al.** *A guide to the responsible service of alcohol.* Toronto, Addiction Research Foundation, 1986.

165. **Franklin, A.** *Pub drinking and the licensed trade*. Bristol, University of Bristol School for Advanced Urban Studies, 1985.

166. *Drinking and driving. A guide for all coach, minibus and taxi operators*. Birmingham, Royal Society for the Prevention of Accidents, 1986.

167. *Drinking and driving. A guide for publicans, hoteliers, restaurateurs and other purveyors of alcohol*. Birmingham, Royal Society for the Prevention of Accidents, 1986.

168. *Drinking and driving. A guide for all organisers of young people's groups*. Birmingham, Royal Society for the Prevention of Accidents, 1986.

169. *Drinking and driving. A guide for employers and employees*. Birmingham, Royal Society for the Prevention of Accidents, 1986.

170. *Drinking and driving. A guide for all organisers of voluntary groups*. Birmingham, Royal Society for the Prevention of Accidents, 1986.

171. **Yates, F. et al.** *Drinking in two North-East towns: a survey of the natural setting for prevention*. Newcastle, Centre for Alcohol and Drug Studies, 1984.

172. **Wood, D.** *Beliefs about alcohol*. London, Health Education Council, 1985 (Research Report No. 5).

173. **Farrell, E.** *Marketing research for local health promotion*. London, Health Education Council, 1986 (Research Report No. 7).

174. **Tether, P.** Prevention of alcohol-related problems. The local dimension. *In*: Stockwell, T. & Clement, S., ed. *Helping the problem drinker. New initiatives in community care*. London, Croom Helm, 1988, pp. 275–298.

175. **Rootman, I. & Moser, J., ed.** *Community response to alcohol-related problems. Report on Phase I of a World Health Organization project*. Geneva, World Health Organization, 1983.

176. **Rootman, I., ed.** *Community response to alcohol-related problems. Report on Phase II of a World Health Organization project*. Geneva, World Health Organization, 1983.

177. **Heather, N.** Change without therapists: the use of self-help manuals by problem drinkers. *In*: Miller, W.R. & Heather, N., ed. *Treating addictive behaviours: processes of change*. New York, Plenum Press, 1986.

178. **Heather, N. et al.** Evaluation of a self-help manual for media-recruited problem drinkers: six month follow-up results. *British journal of clinical psychology*, **25**: 19–34 (1986).

179. **Saunders, W. & Kershaw, P.** Spontaneous remission from alcoholism — a community study. *British journal of addiction*, **74**: 251–266 (1979).

180. **Heather, N.** Minimal treatment interventions for problem drinkers. *In*: Edwards, G. *Current issues in clinical psychology.* London, Plenum Press, 1986.

181. **Skinner, H.A. & Holt, S.** Early intervention for alcohol problems. *Journal of the Royal College of General Practitioners*, **33**: 787–791 (1983).

182. **Catford, J.C. & Nutbeam, D.** Prevention in practice: what Wessex general practitioners are doing. *British medical journal*, **288**: 832–834 (1984).

183. **Wallace, P.G. & Haines, A.P.** General practitioners and health promotion: what patients think. *British medical journal*, **289**: 534–536 (1984).

184. **Aasland, O.G. et al.** Alcohol problems in general practice. *British journal of addiction*, **82**: 197–201 (1987).

185. **Babar, T.F. et al.** Alcohol-related problems in the primary health care setting: a review of early intervention strategies. *British journal of addiction*, **81**: 23–46 (1986).

186. **Anderson, P.** Early intervention in general practice. *In*: Stockwell, T. & Clement, S., ed. *Helping the problem drinker*. London, Croom Helm, 1988.

187. **Ford, A.F.** *Alcohol survey — primary care level workers' case loads 1982–84*. Newcastle-upon-Tyne, Northumberland Alcohol Services, 1984.

188. **Trell, E.** Community-based preventive medical department for individual risk factor assessment and intervention in an urban population. *Preventive medicine*, **12**: 397–402 (1983).

189. *Conditions of work digest*. Geneva, International Labour Office, 1987, Vol. 6, pp. 1–243.

190. **Shaw, S. et al.** *Responding to drinking problems*. London, Croom Helm, 1978.

191. **Clement, S.** The Salford experiment: an account of the community alcohol team approach. *In*: Stockwell, T. & Clement, S., ed. *Helping the problem drinker*. London, Croom Helm, 1988.

192. **Spratley, T.** Consultancy as part of community alcohol team (CAT) work. *In*: Stockwell, T. & Clement, S., ed. *Helping the problem drinker*. London, Croom Helm, 1988.

193. **Chick, J.** Early intervention in the general hospital. *In*: Stockwell, T. & Clement, S., ed. *Helping the problem drinker*. London, Croom Helm, 1988.

194. **Emrick, C.D.** A review of psychologically orientated treatments of alcoholism. II. The relative effectiveness of different treatment approaches and the effectiveness of treatment versus no treatment. *Journal of studies on alcohol*, **36**: 88–168 (1975).

195. **Costello, R.M.** Alcoholism treatment and evaluation: collation of two-year follow-up studies. *International journal of addictions*, **10**: 857–867 (1975).

196. **Polich, J.M. et al.** *The course of alcoholism. Four years after treatment.* New York, John Wiley & Sons, 1980.
197. **Orford, J. & Edwards, G.** *Alcoholism.* Oxford, Oxford University Press, 1977 (Maudsley Monographs No. 26).
198. **Miller, W.R. & Hester, R.K.** The effectiveness of treatment techniques: what works and what doesn't. *In:* Cox, M.E., ed. *Treatment and prevention of alcohol problems. A resources manual.* New York, Academic Press, 1985.
199. **Orford, J. & Wawman, T.** *Alcohol detoxification services: a review.* London, H.M. Stationery Office, 1986.
200. **Hashimi, L. et al.** *Problem drinking. Experiments in detoxification.* London, Bedford Square Press, 1925.
201. **Davies, P. & Walsh, D.** *Alcohol problems and alcohol control in Europe.* London, Croom Helm, 1983.
202. **Heather, N. et al., ed.** *The misuse of alcohol.* London, Croom Helm, 1985.
203. **Grant, M. & Ritson, B.** *Alcohol — the prevention debate.* London, Croom Helm, 1983.
204. **Bruun, K. et al.** *Alcohol control policies in public health perspectives.* Forssa, Finnish Foundation for Alcohol Studies, 1975, Vol. 25.
205. **Miller, P.M. & Nirenberg, T.D., ed.** *Prevention of alcohol abuse.* New York, Plenum Press, 1984.
206. **Central Policy Review Staff.** *Alcohol policies in the United Kingdom.* Stockholm, Sociologiska Institutionen, 1982.
207. **Moser, J.** *Problems and programmes related to alcohol and drug dependence in 33 countries.* Geneva, World Health Organization, 1974 (WHO Offset Publication No. 6).
208. **Moser, J.** *Prevention of alcohol-related problems.* Geneva/Toronto, World Health Organization/Addiction Research Foundation, 1980.
209. **Farrell, S.** *Review of national policy measures to prevent alcohol-related problems.* Geneva, World Health Organization, 1985 (unpublished document WHO/MNH/PAD/85.14).
210. **Moser, J., ed.** *Alcohol policies in national health and development planning.* Geneva, World Health Organization, 1985 (WHO Offset Publication No. 89).
211. **Mäkelä, K. et al.** *Alcohol, society and the state. Vol. 1: a comparative study of alcohol control.* Toronto, Addiction Research Foundation, 1981.
212. **Single, E. et al., ed.** *Alcohol, society and the state. Vol. 2: the social history of control policy in seven countries.* Toronto, Addiction Research Foundation, 1981.
213. **Grant, M., ed.** *Alcohol policies.* Copenhagen, WHO Regional Office for Europe, 1985 (WHO Regional Publications, European Series, No. 18).

214. **Grant, M. et al.** *Economics and alcohol.* London, Croom Helm, 1982.
215. **Godfrey, C.** *Factors influencing the consumption of alcohol and tobacco — a review of demand models.* York, Centre for Health Economics, 1986 (Discussion Paper No. 17).
216. **Godfrey, C. & Powell, M.** *Budget strategies for alcohol and tobacco tax in 1987 and beyond.* York, Centre for Health Economics, 1987 (Discussion Paper No. 22).
217. **Maynard, A.** Economic measures in preventing drinking. *In:* Heather, N. et al., ed. *The misuse of alcohol.* London, Croom Helm, 1985.
218. *Macroeconomic model equation and variable listing.* London, H.M. Treasury Department, 1980.
219. **Department of Health and Social Security.** *Drinking sensibly.* London, H.M. Stationery Office, 1981.
220. **McGuinness, T.** An econometric analysis of total demand for alcoholic beverages in the UK, 1956–75. *Journal of industrial economics,* September, pp. 85–109 (1980).
221. **Duffy, J.C. & Plant, M.A.** Scotland's liquor licensing changes: an assessment. *British medical journal,* **292**: 36–39 (1986).
222. **Goddard, E.** *Drinking and attitudes to licensing in Scotland.* London, H.M. Stationery Office, 1986.
223. **van Iwaarden, M.J.** Advertising, alcohol consumption and policy alternatives. *In:* Grant, M. et al., ed. *Economics and alcohol.* London, Croom Helm, 1983.
224. **McGuinness, T.** The demand for beer, spirits and wine in the UK, 1956–1979. *In:* Grant, M. et al., ed. *Economics and alcohol.* London, Croom Helm, 1983.
225. **Strickland, D.E.** Advertising exposure, alcohol consumption and misuse of alcohol. *In:* Grant, M. et al., ed. *Economics and alcohol.* London, Croom Helm, 1983.
226. **Smart, R.J. & Cutler, R.E.** The alcohol advertising ban in British Colombia: problems and effects on beverage consumption. *British journal of addiction,* **71**: 13–21 (1976).
227. **Ogborne, A.C. & Smart, R.G.** Will restrictions on alcohol advertising reduce alcohol consumption? *British journal of addiction,* **75**: 293–296 (1980).
228. *Health education in the prevention of alcohol related problems.* Edinburgh, Scottish Health Education Co-ordinating Committee, 1985.
229. **Plant, M.A. et al.** Evaluation of the Scottish Health Education Unit's 1976 campaign on alcoholism. *Social psychiatry,* **14**: 11–24 (1979).
230. **Thorley, A.** The role of mass media campaigns in alcohol health education. *In:* Heather, N. et al., ed. *The misuse of alcohol.* London, Croom Helm, 1985.

231. **Cavanagh, J. & Clairmonte, F.F.** *Alcoholic beverages: dimensions of corporate power.* London, Croom Helm, 1985.

232. **Single, E.W.** The structure of the alcohol industry as it relates to transportation issues. *Accident analysis and prevention*, **19**: 419–431 (1987).

233. **Booth, M. et al.** The UK alcohol and tobacco industries. *British journal of addiction*, **81**: 825–830 (1986).

234. **Godfrey, C. & Hardman, G.** Employment in the UK alcohol and tobacco industries. *British journal of addiction*, **82**: 1157–1167 (1987).

235. Alcohol problems. *British medical journal*, 1982.

236. **Anderson, P.** Health authority policies for the prevention of alcohol problems. *British journal of addiction*, **84**: 203–209 (1989).

237. **Wilson, J.M.G. & Jungner, G.** *The principles and practice of screening for disease.* Geneva, World Health Organization, 1968 (Public Health Papers No. 34).

238. **Reid, A.L.A. et al.** General practitioners' detection of patients with high alcohol intake. *British medical journal*, **293**: 735–737 (1986).

239. **Streissguth, A.P. et al.** Test-retest reliability assessment of three scales derived from a quantity-frequency-variability assessment of self-reported alcohol consumption. *Annals of the New York Academy of Sciences*, **273**: 458–466 (1976).

240. **Straus, R. & Bacon, S.D.** *Drinking in college.* New York, Yale University Press, 1953.

241. **Barrison, I.G. et al.** Detecting excessive drinking among admissions to a general hospital. *Health trends*, **14**: 80–83 (1982).

242. **Wallace, P.G. et al.** Drinking patterns in general practice patients. *Journal of the Royal College of General Practitioners*, **37**: 354–357 (1987).

243. *That's the limit.* London, Health Education Council, 1983.

244. **Uchalik, D.C.** A comparison of questionnaire and self-monitored reports of alcohol intake in a non-alcoholic population. *Addictive behaviours*, **4**: 409–413 (1979).

245. **Poikolainen, K. et al.** Correlations between biological markers and alcohol intake as measured by diary and questionnaire in men. *Journal of studies on alcohol*, **46**: 223–227 (1985).

246. **Williams, G.D. et al.** Reliability of self-reported alcohol consumption in a general population survey. *Journal of studies on alcohol*, **46**: 223–227 (1985).

247. **Cooke, D.J. & Allan, C.A.** Self-reported alcohol consumption and dissimulation in a Scottish urban sample. *Journal of studies on alcohol*, **44**: 617–629 (1983).

248. **Skinner, H.A. et al.** Lifestyle assessment: applying microcomputers in family practice. *British medical journal*, **290**: 212–214 (1985).

249. **Lucas, R.W. et al.** Psychiatrists and a computer as interrogators of patients with alcohol-related illnesses: a comparison. *British journal of psychiatry*, **131**: 160–167 (1977).

250. **Jellinek, W.M.** Phases in drinking history of alcoholics: analysis of a survey conducted by the official organ of Alcoholics Anonymous. *Quarterly journal of studies on alcohol*, **7**: 1–88 (1946).

251. **Selzer, M.L.** The Michigan Alcoholism Screening Test. The quest for a new diagnostic instrument. *American journal of psychiatry*, **127**: 1653–1658 (1971).

252. **Moore, R.A.** The diagnosis of alcoholism in a psychiatric hospital: a trial of the Michigan Alcoholism Screening Test (MAST). *American journal of psychiatry*, **128**: 1656–1659 (1972).

253. **Pokorny, A.D. et al.** The brief MAST: a shortened version of the Michigan Alcoholism Screening Test. *American journal of psychiatry*, **129**: 342–345 (1972).

254. **Kaplan, H. et al.** Screening tests and self-identification in the detection of alcoholism. *Journal of health and social behaviour*, **15**: 51–60 (1974).

255. **Saunders, W.M. & Kershaw, P.W.** Screening tests for alcoholism — findings from a community study. *British journal of addiction*, **75**: 37–41 (1980).

256. **Kristenson, H. & Trell, E.** Indicators of alcohol consumption: comparisons between a questionnaire (Mm-MAST), interviews and serum γ-glutamyl transferase (GGT) in a health survey of middle-aged males. *British journal of addiction*, **77**: 2297–2304 (1982).

257. **Nicol, E.F. & Ford, M.J.** Use of the Michigan Alcoholism Screening Test in general practice. *Journal of the Royal College of General Practitioners*, **36**: 409–410 (1986).

258. **Hotch, D.F. et al.** Use of the self-administered Michigan Alcoholism Screening Test in a family practice center. *Journal of family practice*, **17**: 1021–1026 (1983).

259. **Gibbs, L.E.** Validity and reliability of the Michigan Alcoholism Screening Test: a review. *Drug and alcohol dependence*, **12**: 279–285 (1983).

260. **Mayfield, D. et al.** The CAGE questionnaire: validation of a new alcoholism screening instrument. *American journal of psychiatry*, **131**: 1121–1123 (1974).

261. **Bush, B. et al.** Screening for alcohol abuse using the CAGE questionnaire. *American journal of medicine*, **82**: 231–235 (1986).

262. Wiseman, S.M. et al. Assessment of drinking patterns in general practice. *Journal of the Royal College of General Practitioners*, **36**: 231–235 (1986).
263. Wilkins, R.H. *The hidden alcoholic in general practice*. London, Elek Science, 1974.
264. Feuerlein, W. et al. Diagnosis of alcoholism: the Munich Alcoholism Test (MALT). *Currents in alcoholism*, **3**: 137–147 (1980).
265. LeGo, P.M. *Le dépistage précoce et systématique du buveur excessif*. Paris, Département d'alcoologie thérapeutique de Riom Laboratoires, 1976.
266. Babor, T.F. et al. *AUDIT. The Alcohol Use Disorders Identification Test: guidelines for use in primary health care*. Geneva, World Health Organization, 1989 (unpublished document WHO/MNH/DAT/89.4).
267. Saunders, J.B. & Aasland, O.G. AUDIT M the World Health Organization screening instrument for harmful and hazardous alcohol consumption. *British journal of addiction* (in press).
268. Kristenson, H. et al. Serum γ-glutamyl transferase: statistical distribution in a middle-aged male population and evaluation of alcohol habits in individuals with elevated levels. *Preventive medicine*, **9**: 108–119 (1980).
269. Kristenson, H. et al. Serum γ-glutamyl transferase in screening and continuous control of heavy drinking middle-aged men. *American journal of epidemiology*, **114**: 862–872 (1981).
270. Kristenson, H. et al. Serum ferritin, γ-glutamyl transferase and alcohol consumption in healthy middle-aged men. *Drug and alcohol dependence*, **8**: 43–50 (1981).
271. Kristenson, H. et al. Convictions for drunkenness or drunken driving, sick absenteeism and morbidity in middle-aged males with different levels of serum γ-glutamyl transferase. *Preventive medicine*, **11**: 403–416 (1982).
272. Petersson, B. et al. Comparison of γ-glutamyl transferase and other health screening tests in average middle-aged males, heavy drinkers and alcohol non-users. *Scandinavian journal of clinical laboratory investigation*, **43**: 141–149 (1983).
273. Petersson, B. et al. Comparison of γ-glutamyl transferase and questionnaire test as alcohol indicators in different risk groups. *Drug and alcohol dependence*, **11**: 279–286 (1983).
274. Petersson, B. et al. Screening and intervention for alcohol-related disease in middle-aged men: the Malmö Preventive Programme. *In*: Ciba Foundation Symposium 110. *The value of preventive medicine*. London, Pitman, 1985, pp. 143–155.
275. Chick, J. et al. Mean cell volume and γ-glutamyl transpeptidase as markers of drinking in working men. *Lancet*, **1**: 1249–1251 (1981).

276. **Stockwell, T. et al.** The Severity of Alcohol Dependence Questionnaire: its use, reliability and validity. *British journal of addiction*, **78**: 145–155 (1983).

277. **Stockwell, T. et al.** The development of a questionnaire to measure severity of alcohol dependence. *British journal of addiction*, **74**: 79–87 (1979).

278. **Potamianos, G.** The use of the Severity of Alcohol Dependence Questionnaire (SADQ) on a sample of problem drinkers presenting at a district general hospital. *Alcohol*, **1**: 441–445 (1984).

279. **Skinner, H.A. et al.** Lifestyle assessment: just asking makes a difference. *British medical journal*, **290**: 214–216 (1985).

280. **Fullard, E. et al.** Facilitating prevention in primary care. *British medical journal*, **289**: 1585–1587 (1984).

281. **Wallace, P. & Haines, A.** Use of a questionnaire in general practice to increase the recognition of problem drinkers. *British medical journal*, **290**: 1949–1953 (1985).

282. **Skinner, H.A. et al.** Early identification of alcohol abuse. 1. Critical issues and psychosocial indicators for a composite index. *Journal of the Canadian Medical Association*, **124**: 1141–1152 (1981).

283. **Holt, S. et al.** Early identification of alcohol abuse. 2. Clinical and laboratory indicators. *Journal of the Canadian Medical Association*, **124**: 1279–1299 (1981).

284. **Clare, A.W.** How good is treatment? *In*: Edwards, G. & Grant, M., ed. *Alcoholism: new knowledge and new responses*. London, Croom Helm, 1977.

285. **Annis, H.M.** Is inpatient rehabilitation of the alcoholic cost-effective? *Advances in alcohol and substance abuse*, **5**: 175–190 (1986).

286. **Rundell, O.H. et al.** Practical benefit/cost analysis for alcoholism programmes. *Alcoholism: clinical and experimental research*, **5**: 497–508 (1981).

287. **Russell, M.A.H. et al.** Effect of general practitioners' advice against smoking. *British medical journal*, **2**: 231–235 (1979).

288. **Jamrozik, K. et al.** Controlled trial of three different smoking interventions in general practice. *British medical journal*, **288**: 1499–1503 (1985).

289. **Kristenson, H. et al.** Identification and intervention of heavy drinking in middle-aged men: results and follow-up of 24–60 months of long-term study with randomized controls. *Alcoholism: clinical and experimental research*, **7**: 203–209 (1983).

290. **Chick, J. et al.** Counselling problem drinkers in medical wards. *British medical journal*, **290**: 965–967 (1985).

291. **Heather, N.** DRAMS for problem drinkers: the potential of a brief intervention by general practitioners and some evidence of its effectiveness. *In*: Stockwell, T. & Clement, S., ed. *New initiatives in community care*. London, Croom Helm, 1987.

292. **Wallace, P. et al.** Effect of general practitioners' advice to heavy drinkers to reduce their alcohol consumption. *British medical journal*, **297**: 663–668 (1988).

293. **Prochaska, J.O. & Diclemente, C.C.** *The transtheoretical approach: crossing traditional boundaries of therapy*. Homewood, IL, Dow Jones-Irwin, 1985.

294. **Heather, N. & Robertson, I.** *Controlled drinking*. London, Methuen, 1983.

295. **Kanfer, F.H. & Busemeyer, J.R.** The use of problem-solving and decision-making in behaviour therapy. *Clinical psychology review*, **2**: 239–266 (1982).

296. **Kanfer, F.H. & Grimm, L.G.** Managing clinical change. A process model of therapy. *Behaviour modification*, **4**: 419–444 (1980).

297. **Miller, W.R. & Taylor, C.A.** Relative effectiveness of bibliotherapy, individual and group self-control training in the treatment of problem drinkers. *Addictive behaviours*, **5**: 13–24 (1980).

298. **Heather, N.** Minimal treatment interventions for problem drinkers. *In*: Edwards, G. & Gill, M., ed. *Current issues in clinical psychology*. London, Plenum, 1985, Vol. 4.

299. **Stockwell, T.** The Exeter Home Detoxification Project. *In*: Stockwell, T. & Clement, S., ed. *New initiatives in community care*. London, Croom Helm, 1987.

300. **Marlatt, G.A. & George, W.H.** Relapse prevention: introduction and overview of the model. *British journal of addiction*, **79**: 261–273 (1984).

301. **Harwin, J.** The excessive drinker and the family: approaches to treatment. *In*: Orford, J. & Harwin, J., ed. *Alcohol and the family*. London, Croom Helm, 1982.

302. **Duckert, F.** *Sex differences in a control training program for alcohol abusers*. Paper presented at the 31st International Institute on the Prevention and Treatment of Alcoholism, Rome, 1985.

303. **Litman, G.** Women and alcohol problems: finding the next questions. *British journal of addiction*, **81**: 601–604 (1986).

304. **Beckman, L.J. & Amaro, H.** Pattern of women's use of alcohol treatment agencies. *In*: Wilsnack, S.C. & Beckman, L., ed. *Alcohol problems in women*. New York, Guildford Press, 1984.

305. **Plant, M.** Alcohol problems. *In*: McPherson, A., ed. *Women's problems in general practice*. Oxford, Oxford University Press, 1986.

306. **James, O.F.W.** The medical consequences of alcoholism in the elderly. *In*: Krasner, M. et al., ed. *Alcohol-related problems: room for manoeuvre*. London, John Wiley, 1984.

307. **Malcolm, M.T.** Problem drinking in the elderly. *In*: Krasner, M. et al., ed. *Alcohol-related problems: room for manoeuvre*. London, John Wiley, 1984.

308. **Mishara, B.L. & Kastenbaum, R.** *Alcohol and old age*. New York, Grune and Stratton, 1980.

309. **Smith, R.** The habitual drunken offender. *In: Alcohol problems*. London, British Medical Journal, 1982.

310. **Edwards, G.** The alcoholic doctor. A case of neglect. *Lancet*, 2: 1297–1298 (1975).

311. **Murray, R.M.** An epidemiological and clinical study of alcoholism in the medical profession. *In*: Madden, J.S. et al., ed. *Aspects of alcohol and drug dependence*. London, Pitman Medical, 1980.

312. **Hore, B.D.F. & Plant, M.A.** *Alcohol problems in employment*. London, Croom Helm, 1981.

313. **Anderson, P.** Alcohol consumption of undergraduates at Oxford University. *Alcohol and alcoholism*, **19**: 77–84 (1984).

314. **Sorensen, T.I.A. et al.** Prospective evaluation of alcohol abuse and alcoholic liver injury in men as predictors of development of cirrhosis. *Lancet*, **2**: 241–244 (1984).

315. **Brunt, P.W. et al.** Studies in alcoholic liver disease in Britain. *Gut*, **15**: 52–58 (1974).

316. **Robinson, D. & Morrissey, M.** *The management of alcohol-related problems in general practice*. Paper presented at the WHO Scientific Working Group on the Management of Alcohol-related Problems in General Practice, London, 1984.

317. **Anderson, P.** Managing alcohol problems in general practice. *British medical journal*, **290**: 1873–1875 (1985).

318. **Thom, B. & Tellez, C.** A difficult business: detecting and managing alcohol problems in general practice. *British journal of addiction*, **81**: 405–418 (1986).

319. **Clement, S.** The identification of alcohol-related problems by general practitioners. *British journal of addiction*, **81**: 257–264 (1986).

320. **Cartwright, A.K.J.** The attitudes of helping agents towards the alcoholic client: the influence of experience support, training and self-esteem. *British journal of addiction*, **75**: 413–431 (1980).

321. **Anderson, P. & Clement, C.** The AAPPQ revisited. The management of general practitioners' attitudes to alcohol problems. *British journal of addiction*, **82**: 753–760 (1987).

322. **Gray, J.A.M.** Continuing medical education: retooling and renaissance. *Lancet*, **1**: 1261–1262 (1986).

323. **Department of Health and Social Security.** Alcohol-related problems in undergraduate medical education. A survey of English medical schools. *Journal of medical education*, **58**: 316–321 (1983).

324. **Clare, A.W.** Alcohol education and the medical student. *Alcohol and alcoholism*, **19**: 291–296 (1984).

325. **Pokorny, A.D. & Solomon, J.** A follow-up survey of drug abuse and alcoholism teaching in medical schools. *Journal of medical education*, **60**: 618–626 (1985).

326. **Hanlon, M.J.** A review of the recent literature relating to the training of medical students in alcoholism. *Journal of medical education*, **60**: 618–626 (1985).

327. **Ashby, M.J. et al.** *Alcohol- and drug-related problems.* Toronto, University of Toronto, 1987.

328. **Association of University Teachers in General Practice.** *Undergraduate medical education in general practice.* London, Royal College of General Practitioners, 1984 (Occasional Paper No. 28).

329. *Alcohol-related problems in higher professional and postgraduate medical education.* London, Department of Health and Social Security, 1987.

330. **Haynes, B.R. et al.** A critical appraisal of the efficacy of continuing medical education. *Journal of the American Medical Association*, **251**: 61–64 (1985).

331. **Gray, J.A.M.** Continuing education: what techniques are effective. *Lancet*, **2**: 447–448 (1986).

332. **Inui, T.S. et al.** Improved outcomes in hypertension after physician tutorials: a controlled trial. *Annals of internal medicine*, **84**: 646–651 (1976).

333. *Drug use and misuse. Group leaders' pack.* Milton Keynes, The Open University, 1987, p. 576.

334. **Heller, T. et al, ed.** *Drug use and misuse.* Chichester, John Wiley & Sons, 1987.

335. **Anderson, P. et al.** *Alcohol — a practical guide.* Oxford, Oxford University Press, 1988.

336. **Devenyi, P. & Saunders, S.J.** *Physicians' handbook for medical management of alcohol- and drug-related problems.* Toronto, Addiction Research Foundation, 1986.

337. **Bain, D. & Taylor, L.** *Counselling skills for alcoholism treatment services.* Toronto, Addiction Research Foundation, 1981.

338. **Fullard, E. et al.** Promoting prevention in primary care: controlled trial of low-technology, low-cost approach. *British medical journal*, **294**: 1080–1082 (1987).

339. **National Institute of Medicine.** *Alcoholism, alcohol abuse and related problems: opportunities for research.* Washington, National Academy Press, 1980.

340. *Report of the second meeting of investigators in the WHO collaborative project on identification and treatment of persons with harmful alcohol consumption.* Geneva, World Health Organization, 1984 (unpublished document).

341. **Skog, O.-J.** Norway: National Institute for Alcohol Research. *British journal of addiction,* **10**: 1073–1079 (1987).

342. **Wald, I. et al.** Poland. *British journal of addiction,* **81**: 729–734 (1988).

343. **Mäkelä, K.** The Finnish Foundation for Alcohol Studies and the Social Research Institute of Alcohol Studies. *British journal of addiction,* **83**: 141–148 (1988).

344. **Bruun, K. & Rosenquist, P.** Nordic countries. *British journal of addiction,* **80**: 245–253 (1985).

345. **Walsh, D.** Ireland. *British journal of addiction,* **82**: 747–751 (1987).

346. **Glass, I.** England, Wales and Northern Ireland. *British journal of addiction,* **81**: 197–215 (1986).

347. **Robinson, D. & Maynard, A.** Hull-York, UK. *British journal of addiction,* **82**: 1185–1190 (1987).

348. **Heather, N.** Addictive Behaviour Research Group: University of Dundee. *British journal of addiction,* **82**: 1301–1305 (1987).

349. **Feuerlein, W. & Kufner, H.** Federal Republic of Germany. *British journal of addiction,* **81**: 613–619 (1986).

350. **Plant, M.A. & Plant, M.L.** Scotland. *British journal of addiction,* **81**: 17–21 (1986).

351. **Kiianman, K.** Research Laboratories of the Finnish State Alcohol Company, Alko Ltd. (Biomedical Department). *British journal of addiction,* **82**: 961–969 (1987).

352. **Anokhina, I.P. et al.** USSR. *British journal of addiction,* **82**: 23–30 (1987).

353. **Crawford, A.** *Register of United Kingdom Alcohol Research, 1985–1986.* Edinburgh, University of Edinburgh Alcohol Research Group, 1986.

In many parts of Europe alcohol consumption
has risen considerably over the past 25–30 years,
and this has been matched by a huge increase
in alcohol-related problems. Many European countries
see this as a major public health problem,
second only to cigarette smoking.

The approach of WHO to this question is to emphasize
the importance of a response embedded in the community
and the need for early recognition,
rather than specialist treatment.
WHO has also suggested ways of using reporting systems
or other strategies for small-scale monitoring,
implying that early recognition is possible
and that nipping the problem in the bud
will prevent further damage.

The book first examines the part played by alcohol
in communities and in individual lives,
and discusses the balance between the factors
that encourage drinking and those that discourage it.
It then goes on to catalogue the harm that can result
from the use of alcohol, to discuss the resources available
for preventing and managing alcohol problems,
and to list ways of promoting health
and preventing alcohol problems.
Finally, the book suggests a structure for ascertaining
and categorizing the alcohol-related risks for individuals
seen in primary care, and ways of informing, advising
and helping people in different categories.

ISBN 92 890 1123 8   Price: Sw.fr. 26.-